Praise for *The Tapping Solution for Parents, Children & Teenagers*

Contrary to popular belief, a parent's primary role is to provide spiritual mentorship and support. But how? This treasure trove of a text provides exactly the tools you need to heal, protect and find balance—for yourself and your little ones.

—Kelly Brogan, MD, Holistic psychiatrist and author of the
New York Times bestseller *A Mind of Your Own*

It has been said that the wounds of the 8th grade have the half life of uranium. In truth, many people carry the wounds and shame of their childhood and schooling right on into adulthood and then pass them on to their children. But it doesn't have to be this way. There is a scientifically based method that changes the way the mind and body respond to stress... transforming it into empowerment and lifelong skills for living well.

In The Tapping Solution for Parents, Children & Teenagers, *Nick Ortner gives you all the tools you need to help you and your kids live a healthier, more stress-resilient life. I also happen to know Nick and his wonderful extended family. All of them are living proof that this practical approach works. And it's at your fingertips. Every parent needs this book!*

—Christiane Northrup, MD, Author of the *New York Times* bestsellers
Goddesses Never Age and *Women's Bodies, Women's Wisdom*

I can't think of a better resource to have on hand when raising children than this book!

Whether you and your child are dealing with social anxiety, fears and phobias, bullying, or the heartbreaking loss of a first love, The Tapping Solution for Parents, Children & Teenagers *will provide you with a simple, yet powerful tool to turn pain and stress into peace and sanity in no time. This book is a must-have manual for every parent!*

—Cheryl Richardson, *New York Times* best-selling author of *Take Time for Your Life*

Too many of our children are anxious, stressed and overwhelmed. Too many are feeling lost and hopeless. The Tapping Solution for Parents, Children & Teenagers *may be just what they and their parents need to bring their lives back in balance. This book gives me hope about our collective future.*

—Kris Carr, *New York Times* best-selling author (and EFT lover)

If you're human, you most likely experienced a traumatic event in your childhood. Unfortunately, most of us grew up without any way of processing, communicating and releasing these painful events.

It doesn't need to be this way for our kids. Nick Ortner has a breakthrough technique that your child can use to recalibrate and empower themselves in those dark moments, and he is going to teach you how to bring it into your daily life.

This book is a must-read for parents and kids of all ages—consider it first aid for your child's self-esteem and mental wellness. As a father of two young boys, I highly recommend it!

—Nick Polizzi, founder of The Sacred Science

More Praise for *The Tapping Solution for Parents, Children & Teenagers*

In a time where video games and searching the internet are the number-one activities for beating stress amongst our teens, there is a need for something more effective.

—Peta Stapleton, PhD, Author of *EFT for Teens* and *Tapping in the Classroom*

The two hardest things about being a parent are: How can we take care of ourselves when there are others who rely on us being present, and wondering if we're going to do something wrong to mess them up for life?

Nick's work has helped our family learn the tools to help lessen the worry and fear around raising kids. We've used these techniques for ourselves to address our fears of being parents and to calm ourselves down when we're on the edge. We've also used Tapping with our children to help our son relax when he's having a tantrum and even to help our daughter with toilet training!

We highly, highly recommend this book!

—Kevin and Annmarie Gianni, Founders of Annmarie Gianni Skin Care

The most important responsibility nature bestows on every new parent is to raise offspring who are happy, healthy and able to contribute to and advance their culture. This challenge has never been greater than it is today.

Fortunately, we have at our disposal powerful practices that were not available to our parents or any generation before them.

Nick Ortner brings some of the most potent of these tools to every parent and child who wishes to learn them, and he offers these resources in a wonderfully practical and accessible format.

—Donna Eden and David Feinstein, Co-authors of *The Promise of Energy Psychology* and *The Energies of Love*

The Tapping Solution

for

Parents, Children & Teenagers

Also by Nick Ortner

The Tapping Solution

The Tapping Solution for Pain Relief

The Tapping Solution for Manifesting Your Greatest Self

The Big Book of Hugs: A Barkley the Bear Story

All of the above are available at your local bookstore,
or may be ordered by visiting:

Hay House USA: www.hayhouse.com®
Hay House Australia: www.hayhouse.com.au
Hay House UK: www.hayhouse.co.uk
Hay House India: www.hayhouse.co.in

The Tapping Solution for Parents, Children & Teenagers

How to Let Go of Excessive Stress, Anxiety and Worry, and Raise Happy, Healthy, Resilient Families

NICK ORTNER

HAY HOUSE, INC.
Carlsbad, California • New York City
London • Sydney • Johannesburg
Vancouver • New Delhi

Copyright © 2018 by Nicolas Ortner

Published and distributed in the United States by: Hay House, Inc.: www.hayhouse.com®
Published and distributed in Australia by: Hay House Australia Pty. Ltd.: www.hayhouse.com.au
Published and distributed in the United Kingdom by: Hay House UK, Ltd.: www.hayhouse.co.uk
Distributed in Canada by: Raincoast Books: www.raincoast.com
Published in India by: Hay House Publishers India: www.hayhouse.co.in

Project editor: Alison Partridge
Cover design: Julie Rosenberger
Interior design: Alex Head/Draft Lab LLC
Tapping Points illustrations: Courtesy of the author
Tapping Tree illustration: © Rachelle Meyer, www.rachellemeyer.com

Library of Congress Cataloging-in-Publication Data

Names: Ortner, Nick, date, author.
Title: The tapping solution for parents, children & teenagers : how to let go
   of excessive stress, anxiety and worry and raise happy, healthy, resilient
   families / Nick Ortner.
Other titles: Tapping solution for parents, children and teenagers
Description: 1st edition. | Carlsbad, California : Hay House, Inc., 2018. |
   Includes index.
Identifiers: LCCN 2017050491 | ISBN 9781401956066 (alk. paper)
Subjects: LCSH: Emotional Freedom Techniques. | Mind and body therapies. |
   Stress (Psychology) | Anxiety. | Self-care, Health.
Classification: LCC RC489.E45 O783 2018 | DDC 616.89/1--dc23 LC record available at https://lccn.
loc.gov/2017050491

ISBN: 978-1-4019-5606-6

10 9 8 7 6 5 4 3 2
1st edition, March 2018

Printed in the United States of America

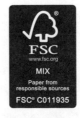
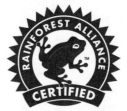

Contents

Introduction

In May of 2015, one of my biggest and most important dreams came true. During the peaceful hours of the late afternoon, my beautiful wife, Brenna, gave birth to our first child. Nearly three years into our marriage, we were officially parents!

In the months that followed, we had our share of long nights and exhausting days. Like all new parents, we were awoken at all hours to feed, change and soothe our baby girl. Time and time again, I would catch myself groaning at the sound of her crying at 3 AM, only to realize that feeding her and rocking her back to sleep was hardly a burden. Sure, the disrupted sleep sometimes felt trying, but caring for her was amazing, heartwarming and profoundly fulfilling. That time and effort was also an integral part of being something I'd always wanted to be—a dad.

As days turned into weeks and then months, I began thinking about the thousands of parents I'd worked with over the past ten-plus years. My mind began replaying the profound transformations so many of them had experienced as a result of Tapping, also known as EFT. I recalled repeatedly how those changes had elevated their entire life experiences, including their experiences as parents.

At the same time, I began thinking back on who I was and how I felt before stumbling upon Tapping back in 2003. I remembered the heavy load of negative emotions and limiting beliefs I too carried before I began Tapping myself.

Thanks to these only sometimes coherent mental ramblings, I was once again humbled by gratitude. Without Tapping, I can say for sure that my first experiences of parenting would have been tainted by my own stress and my personal limiting beliefs. But instead, because of my years of Tapping both on myself and with millions of people around the world, I was filled with overwhelming love and joy as I held our sweet, bubbly little girl in my arms.

For me, and for so many people I've worked with, Tapping has been nothing short of life-changing. What more important service could I provide than to share this technique with the people—namely parents—whose job I myself was just beginning to understand?

And so, the seeds of this book were planted.

In the many months that followed, I worked with a group of parents and witnessed yet again how profoundly even a little bit of Tapping can transform, expand and uplift our experience around parenting.

Given how busy parents are, I set out to create a short program that required minimal time and effort. There were no worksheets or journaling assignments, just the option to use Tapping if and when participating parents were able.

In the end we accepted about 50 parents into that program, which we called *The Tapping Solution for Parents Group*. It consisted of four weekly one-hour calls, Tapping on issues related to parenting.

It was one of the most "bare bones" programs I've ever offered, but once again, I was thrilled and amazed by the incredible transformations that took place in that group.

Hearing parents' stories, I was struck by the breadth and depth of the challenges that their children were facing. Wanting to help not just parents, but entire families, I sought out stories of children using Tapping, and was blown away by what I heard. In this book, you will read a wide variety of real-life scenarios of people who used Tapping to benefit their lives and those around them.

As you can perhaps tell from the sheer volume of pages now in your hands, this book grew quickly. What began as a guide for parents to shed stress and transform their experience around parenting became a two-part book that includes a large section about how to tap with children.

In Part 1, which includes Chapters 1–7, I share an accessible, easy-to-follow Tapping process for parents. This is where you will let go of excessive stress, anxiety, worry and overwhelm, and in so doing, transform your everyday experience around parenting.

Again, I intentionally created a process that provides optimal results in the least amount of time. As a result, you'll notice shorter chapters, along with plenty of opportunities to tap.

I urge you to use this section as your time out, a gift from you to yourself. It can and will change your experience around parenting if you follow it—and if you do the Tapping!

Part 2 of this book is a different animal altogether. It's essentially a reference book that you can use to tap with your child on issues s/he may face now and in the future.

To make this section as useful as possible, I focused on school-aged children, beginning in kindergarten and extending through high school. Due to their expanding awareness of themselves and the world around them, this is the age range when children stand to benefit the most from Tapping. It's also when kids can learn how to tap by themselves.

Part 2 begins with a chapter on how to tap with kids of different age groups, and each subsequent chapter then functions as a stand-alone guide on how to tap on a specific issue. Every one of the sections within these chapters includes Tapping scripts for you and your child, and the majority of them also offer stories of children who have used Tapping to shift their experience around that particular issue.

The list of topics in Part 2 covers a wide range of common challenges children face today, including ADD and ADHD, Allergies and Asthma, Anger, Bullying, Anxiety, Physical Pain, Shame, Grief, as well as issues related to Divorce, Relationships, Sleep, Trauma, Nightmares, Young Love and much more. And even if the specific problem your child is facing isn't found in these pages, in Part 2 you'll find ideas about how to use Tapping with your child on what s/he is experiencing.

Given what a huge and important role teachers and school counselors play in our children's lives, I also wanted to provide Tapping resources for them. What I heard repeatedly, though, was that regulations and time limitations often prevented schools from adopting practices like Tapping. Rather than providing lengthy written content, I instead wrote an Addendum for teachers and school staff interested in bringing Tapping into their schools and classrooms. These pages are further supplemented through online resources created to help teachers, school administrators and counselors propose and implement Tapping in schools.

I am so excited to offer this book to you. I can't imagine a more important and deserving audience than you, the parents and caretakers whose immense everyday contributions are shaping our world and our future.

I hope you'll join me on this beautiful journey, and, along with millions of others, use Tapping to transform and recreate your everyday experiences around parenting.

Nick Ortner

PART ONE

Cultivating Peace, Becoming Present

Chapter 1

Kids, the Brain and Stress

Picture Jenny, a 5th grader who is standing at the front of the class about to read her writing assignment aloud. As she looks down at the page, then up at the faces of her classmates, time slows. Her heartbeat grows louder and faster.

She's nervous, *very* nervous, and more than anything, she wants to escape.

Jenny looks over at her teacher, who nods at her to begin reading. Jenny does as instructed, but before finishing the first sentence, she stumbles and mispronounces a word. The entire class erupts in what sounds to Jenny like the whole world laughing at her. Even the teacher suppresses a giggle before standing up to ask the class to quiet down.

Jenny is shocked and bewildered, unsure what to do and unable to move. She wishes that she could run straight home, but instead finishes as quickly as she can, reading very quietly for fear of getting laughed at again.

Many of us have had "Jenny" moments, big and small events from our childhood where we felt humiliated, afraid and alone. Once we become parents, a story like this may strike us very differently. We wonder and worry, *What dam-*

age will an event like this do—to Jenny's self-esteem, her feelings about school, her friends, her teacher? And what should I, as her parent or teacher, do—or not do—to help her handle experiences like this?

We feel conflicted, wanting both to protect Jenny and to give her the tools she needs to develop on her own. At times we may also take on her emotions and feel overwhelmed by them.

In the midst of managing our own experience, we wonder how we can best support our children. Above all we want to make days like Jenny's feel less challenging. We want her to experience self-esteem, joy and excitement about her life. We want her academic, social and emotional experiences to inspire positive growth and evolution.

Yet we ourselves often feel consumed by daily life, sandwiched between pressure from work, finances, family, not to mention the endless cultural pressure to be the "perfect" parent. How can we help her, when we're struggling ourselves? How can we best help Jenny, and perhaps also ourselves, to thrive, now and in the future?

One important place to start is by addressing one of the main issues that's stopping our children from thriving, and that's stress. It can seem like an unusual starting point, given that our conversations around stress typically focus on adults. Yet the results of recent research around stress and kids are, to put it mildly, shocking.

- According to the American Psychological Association, almost one-third of kids suffer from stress that manifests physically in the form of headaches, stomachaches, and more.[1]

- A Stanford University study found that the number of kids ages 7–17 who are suffering from depression more than doubled between 1985 and 2001.[2]

These trends around kids and stress don't just seem to be continuing. They seem to be worsening.

KIDS AND THE STRESS RESPONSE

Standing in front of her class, Jenny's heart began to race. Her face felt hot, and her hands clammy. The stress Jenny was feeling wasn't just in her head; it was also in her body. Before she'd even said a word, an almond-shaped part of her mid-brain called the **amygdala** received a danger signal. Immediately her body was flooded with a mixture of powerful hormones, including adrenaline and cortisol, the latter often known as the stress hormone, which put her whole body on high alert.

As a result of the cortisol now flooding her body, several "non-essential" functions, including digestion and the creative center of her brain, promptly shut down. While some of her physical senses may have temporarily heightened, her ability to problem-solve and focus on schoolwork had been temporarily sidelined.

This process, which is known as the *stress response* or *"fight or flight,"* happened in a matter of seconds without her conscious awareness.

While this stress response would naturally subside if Jenny had a positive experience, in Jenny's case it intensified. Instead of relaxing into the experience of reading aloud to her class, Jenny panicked when her class laughed at her misread word.

As a result of their laugher, Jenny's stress response grew more pronounced, instantaneously morphing into the "freeze response." In Jenny's case, that translated into feeling like she couldn't move or respond in any way to the class's laughter.

This "freeze response" is a defensive mechanism, an emotional and physical response to panic or extreme stress that we also see in nature. For instance, opossums are known for "freezing" when they're under potential attack from predators. By "playing opossum," as it's often called, they appear to be dead already, and as a result, predators may become disinterested and leave. The opossum can then spring back into action and flee to safety.

Since Jenny is unable to escape to safety, her hands begin to tremble, and her stomach feels queasy. In an attempt to protect her from future experiences like this one, her brain also begins transforming, creating neural pathways that associate public speaking with danger.

Throughout the rest of the day, Jenny replays that moment in her head over and over again. Each time she does, her shame intensifies. *How could I be so stupid?* she thinks. By the time the school day ends, Jenny has relived that moment hundreds of times. At dinner, her stomach is so upset that she barely eats, and asks her parents if she can go to bed early.

So what happened that turned this one experience into the cause of so much distress?

Every time Jenny replayed the moment when she was laughed at, her body re-initiated the stress response. Each time this pattern was repeated–1) remembering reading to the class and getting laughed at, then 2) initiating the stress response—her brain reinforced the neural pathways that associate public speaking with danger. These changes are made possible by the brain's ability to "reorganize itself by forming new neural connections throughout life," a characteristic known as *neuroplasticity*.[3]

As a result of these newly organized neural pathways, reliving her public speaking fiasco has become as vivid and intense as her actual public speaking experience was. With this neural pathway being continually strengthened by repeated memory recall, just thinking about public speaking is enough to cause her body to be hijacked by the stress response. In addition to shutting down her digestion (which, in her case, translates into a lack of appetite), this stress response also makes her more susceptible to physical pain—hence, the stomachache that sends her to bed earlier than usual.

THE STRESS RESPONSE IMPRINT

Fast-forward two years, and Jenny seems like a happy, normal 7th grader.

She's got friends, does well in school, and enjoys team sports. Sitting in class at the start of the year, however, Jenny is overcome by terror when her teacher explains that each student in the class will be required to read their essays out loud. Jenny doesn't mind writing the essay—she actually enjoys that part—but reading it aloud? That's a different story!

Just the thought of it makes her break out in a sweat.

She can't live through being laughed at again. Feeling increasingly panicked, she talks to her teacher after class and asks if she can write an extra essay instead of reading her one essay aloud. He says no, and tells her not to be afraid. She's a good student. She'll be fine.

Jenny spends the next three weeks in a state of panic. She has an unusually hard time writing her essay, doesn't sleep well (nightmares), and is less social at school. She's consumed by her nervousness, and feels increasingly desperate to get out of the requirement to read her essay aloud.

When the day arrives, Jenny is exhausted and stressed out. During her presentation she makes a point of speaking very slowly and quietly, but she still skips a few words, then an entire paragraph, and soon notices her classmates passing notes and making faces while she's speaking.

Once again, she's failed.

Once again, she spends the rest of that day, and many of the days to come, replaying her disastrous performance at the front of the class.

She feels humiliated and ashamed. To make matters worse, a week later she finds out she got a C on her essay and presentation. Usually a B+ student, Jenny is devastated. She decides that she's bad at public speaking. It's a fact, she tells herself, and something she needs to avoid at all costs.

In addition to validating her fear of public speaking, Jenny's most recent experience has once again deepened and strengthened the neural pathways that equate public speaking with danger. Her belief that she is a bad public speaker feels increasingly legitimate. She can't do it, she thinks, so she makes a point of only pursuing activities that allow her to be less visible, like playing in the band or on sports teams where she can blend in.

Jenny's strategy to avoid public speaking works well for a fairly long stretch of years. She manages to do well in grade school, then college. She gets good jobs for several years after graduation. As the years pile up, however, her career seems to slow down prematurely.

Now 32 years old with a family of her own, Jenny is frustrated that she's not getting promoted. She's a hard worker, has great experience and good ideas. When she finally works up the nerve to ask her boss about getting promoted, her boss tells Jenny that her poor presentation skills are holding her back. In order to get promoted, she'll need to be able to step into a leadership position. That means taking on a new level of responsibility, including presenting in front of colleagues, clients and larger groups.

Jenny's fear of public speaking has grown so intense and visceral over the years that she'll do almost anything to avoid speaking to groups.

Even large group meetings are terrifying. She's beginning to realize that her career dreams will remain out of reach because of it, but she's stuck. Her fear of public speaking isn't just emotional. It's also physical. On the rare occasions when she speaks in a group, her voice shakes, she gets clammy hands, and her stomach begins to churn. Every single time she's tried public speaking, she's failed.

What can she do?

More importantly, what could have been possible if she'd been given a way to release her stress, fear and shame around public speaking after being laughed at in 5th or 7th grade?

THE BRAIN'S "NEGATIVITY BIAS"

Before we look at how to halt the pattern of stress that's preventing Jenny from being a successful public speaker, it helps to understand the human brain's "negativity bias."

For our own protection, the brain evolved to assume the worst—it's biased toward negativity. In his book *Hardwiring Happiness*, Rick Hanson, PhD, explains this concept in more detail:

"Our ancestors could make two kinds of mistakes:

(1) thinking there was a tiger in the bushes when there wasn't one, and

(2) thinking there was no tiger in the bushes when there actually was one.

The cost of the first mistake was needless anxiety, while the cost of the second one was death.

Consequently, we evolved to make the first mistake a thousand times to avoid making the second mistake even once."

Hanson continues:

"In general the default setting of the brain is to *over*estimate threats, *under*estimate opportunities, and *under*estimate resources both for coping with threats and for fulfilling opportunities. Then we update these beliefs with information that confirms them, while ignoring or rejecting information that doesn't. There are even regions in the amygdala specifically designed to prevent the unlearning of fear, especially from childhood experiences. As a result, we end up preoccupied by threats that are actually smaller or more manageable than we'd feared, while overlooking opportunities that are actually greater than we'd hoped for. In effect, we've got a brain that's prone to 'paper tiger paranoia.'"[4]

We see this "negativity bias" play out in Jenny's story. After that one negative experience in 5th grade, Jenny's fear of speaking in groups became so ingrained that it prevented her from participating in any form of public speaking, and her fear was still limiting her in her 30s. That's her brain's "negativity bias" at work.

To put it another way, because of how our brains have evolved, negative experiences routinely outweigh positive ones.

The psychologist Daniel Kahneman received the Nobel Prize in economics for showing that most people will do more to avoid loss than to benefit from an equivalent gain. In intimate relationships, we typically need at least five positive interactions to counterbalance every negative one. And for people to begin to thrive in life, they usually need positive moments to outweigh negative ones by at least a three-to-one ratio.[5]

> *For people to begin to thrive in life, they usually*
> *need positive moments to outweigh negative*
> *ones by at least a three-to-one ratio.*

So how can we reverse this process, and prevent the stress Jenny experiences in 5th grade from interfering with her success in 7th grade and beyond?

TAPPING INTO THE RELAXATION RESPONSE

The secret to unraveling Jenny's pattern of stress around public speaking lies in the body's opposite response—*the relaxation response.*

In this more positive state of mind, cortisol levels in the body naturally go down. As a result, Jenny can more easily access the creative center of her brain. Her body can once again support healthy digestion and metabolism, among other processes. She's also less susceptible to illness and physical pain from headaches, stomachaches, injuries and more.

The question is, in a case like Jenny's, how can we quickly disrupt the stress response and initiate the relaxation response? There's a growing body of research suggesting that Tapping, or EFT, is a simple but powerful way to do exactly that. In a double-blind study conducted by Dawson Church, PhD, the control group, which received conventional talk therapy, showed only a 14 percent drop in cortisol levels, whereas the Tapping group showed an average decrease of 24 percent, a substantial and important difference. Some study participants experienced a decrease of as much as 50 percent in their cortisol levels. Within both groups, these changes all took place within a one-hour period.[6]

Research has also shown that acupuncture increases endorphin levels in the body. Since Tapping engages the same acupuncture points while also lowering cortisol, it is inferred that Tapping, like acupuncture, allows the body to release the endorphins that then reinforce positive feelings, as well as physical and emotional well-being.

The incredible results that Tapping has demonstrated in relieving stress may be explained, at least in part, by its ability to access what are called meridian channels.

Although awareness of these channels dates back to thousands of years in ancient Chinese medicine, it wasn't until the 1960s that these threadlike, microscopic anatomical structures were first seen on stereomicroscope and electron microscope images. The scans showed tubular structures, 30 to 100 micrometers wide, running up and down the body. Described in a published paper by a North Korean researcher named Kim Bonghan, they are also referred to as "Bonghan channels."[7] As a reference point, one red blood cell is 6 to 8 micrometers wide, so these structures are tiny!

You can think of meridian channels as a fiber-optic network in the body. They carry a large amount of information, mostly electrical and often beyond what the nervous system or chemical systems of the body can carry. By accessing these channels while processing emotions, thoughts and physical conditions like pain, Tapping gets to the root cause of stress more quickly than other stress relief techniques can.

Given that Tapping sends calming, relaxing signals directly to the amygdala, it may also help us to override the brain's negativity bias more rapidly. By using Tapping to neutralize what it thought were threats to its survival—which in Jenny's case was public speaking—we may be able to reprogram the brain to support more positive experiences.

TRANSFORMING JENNY'S FUTURE

Given also what we now know about Tapping and stress, let's take a quick look at Jenny's 5th-grade public speaking experience, and how Tapping could have transformed her future from an earlier age.

In this version of the story, she's just finished her humiliating turn at the front of the class. Her face is burning with shame, and she feels mortified.

That night at home, her parents notice that she seems bothered, and ask her if she wants to talk about anything. She says no, but then at bedtime, she shares what happened in class when she read her essay aloud. As she tells her parents the story, she begins crying. Her parents ask her if she wants to do some Tapping on the experience.

After 10 or so minutes of Tapping on her memory of speaking in front of the class that day, Jenny calms noticeably. She's smiling again, and quickly falls asleep.

Two years later, Jenny again feels a bit nervous about reading her 7th-grade essay aloud to her class, but remembers to tap on her anxiety. During that time, she's able to enjoy writing her essay, and then has a successful speaking experience. Throughout middle and high school, Jenny becomes very involved in theater, regularly using Tapping on performance anxiety, and finds that she loves to perform.

Once out of college, Jenny is able to use her speaking and presentation skills in her career. During the many years that follow, she is given ample opportunity to fulfill her potential and pursue her passion and interests.

What a difference, and all of that from 10 minutes of Tapping in 5th grade!

With that in mind, let's start looking at how powerful this technique can be for kids who have used Tapping in their lives and realized its incredible, lasting benefits.

FROM ANXIOUS TO ACE PERFORMER

When Marla showed up for her singing lesson, she was in a panic.

After spending months practicing her piece, Marla felt sure that she was going to perform poorly on the final singing exam she was due to take the following week. Although a very talented singer, Marla had historically performed poorly in sight singing, which would comprise one entire section of her upcoming final exam.

Sight singing, which is singing a piece on sight without advance preparation, had always been Marla's Achilles' heel, the one part of her singing that she'd been unable to master. If her past history was any indication, her inability to perform in sight singing would hold her back from what might otherwise be a successful singing career.

As she shared her growing sense of panic with her voice teacher, Suzanne, Marla's entire body visibly tensed. Knowing that their practice time together was limited, Suzanne led Marla through several rounds of Tapping on her anxiety about sight singing. After 15 minutes, Marla's anxiety around this issue had nearly vanished. They then moved on, finishing their session by practicing as they normally do. At the end of their time together, Suzanne wished Marla well on the exam.

Two weeks later, Marla returned with her test results. In addition to getting high marks for her aria singing, Marla had done better than ever before in her sight singing! They were among the best scores Marla had ever received.

Years of anxiety, fear and frustration around sight singing had been reversed in just 15 minutes of Tapping!

FROM TEST ANXIETY TO BETTER SLEEP AND MORE... TAPPING REALLY IS FOR *EVERYONE*

Marla is one of countless students—and Suzanne one of countless parents and teachers—who, thanks to Tapping, have broken through past limitations to achieve what previously seemed impossible.

As we've seen in Marla's story, as well as in the positive version of Jenny's story, the transformation often begins with a parent, teacher or caretaker. Had Marla's singing teacher or Jenny's parents been distracted or unsure how to guide a child through Tapping, neither Marla nor Jenny could have experienced the incredible transformation they each did.

That's why the best first step is for you, as a parent or caretaker, to practice Tapping on yourself. So let's start Tapping!

Chapter 2

Quick and Powerful Stress Relief

When parents first learn about Tapping, they often wonder if it will resolve a specific issue their child is having. Maybe they want to help their kids with test anxiety or social issues at school, like bullying, or challenges with siblings, or perhaps coming to grips with their parents' divorce.

My answer is often a resounding yes! Tapping can and does address a long list of specific concerns that relate to children's performance (academic, athletic, artistic and more), social emotional development, as well as their physical health and well-being (migraines, physical pain, stomachaches, ADD, trauma, etc.).

But the most powerful place to begin Tapping is with what you're experiencing right now. If your goal is to use Tapping with your child's anxiety disorder, rest assured, this book will show you how to do that. The fastest way to begin learning how to tap with your child, however, is to take a few minutes to tap on yourself right now, starting with whatever's most bothering you at this exact moment.

It is critical that you have a direct personal experience with Tapping before attempting to share it with your children, or you won't be able to share it with them. So if you're currently stressed out about work, or a fight you had this morning, or physical pain you're experiencing, that's the best place to start.

We'll call that your Most Pressing Issue, or MPI.

> ### TECHNIQUES FOR TAPPING WITH CHILDREN OF ALL AGES
>
> In future chapters we'll also discuss in detail different ways to introduce Tapping to children of different ages. Needless to say, we'll take a very different approach introducing Tapping to a teenager versus a child in elementary school. As I've shared, though, the best and fastest way to help your child is to first get comfortable with Tapping yourself.

DIRECT TAPPING ON WHAT'S BOTHERING YOU NOW

Step 1: Focus on Your Most Pressing Issue (MPI)

Before Tapping, you first need to focus your attention on what's bothering you most. Start with the one issue or problem that feels most pressing at this moment. Then ask yourself, When I think about this issue, what do I feel in my body? Do I feel tension, pain, heat or cold? Do I feel emptiness, numbness or nothingness? It's important to pay attention to feedback from your body. There are no wrong answers here, so just notice your answers, trying to be as specific as possible about your experience.

Step 2: Measure the Intensity

Now that you have a clearer sense of your MPI and of how your body feels when you think of it, give your MPI a number for its intensity on a scale of 0 to 10. This is called the SUDS, or Subjective Units of Distress Scale. When you focus on your MPI, how intense does it feel at this moment? A 10 would be the most intense you can imagine; a 0 would mean you don't feel any intensity at all.

Don't worry about getting the SUDS level exact or "right"—just follow your gut instinct. To see a significant shift, try to start with an MPI that has an intensity rating of 5 or higher. Make a note of the SUDS number for the MPI you will be addressing.

Step 3: Craft Your Setup Statement

With your SUDS level in mind, your next step is to craft what's called the "setup statement." This statement describes and focuses your mind on your MPI. Once you know your setup statement, you can start Tapping.

The basic setup statement might go like this:

Even though I <describe your MPI>, I deeply and completely love and accept myself.

So, for example, you might say, "Even though I'm so worried about my child's test anxiety, I deeply and completely love and accept myself."

Or, "Even though my shoulders tense every time I think about my child's anxiety, I deeply and completely accept myself."

Your setup statement should resonate with what you're experiencing when you begin Tapping. The goal is not to say magic words as if they're the formula that unlocks the door to stress relief, but to say words that have *meaning* to you, so if the basic setup statement doesn't ring true or feel powerful, change it.

Here are a few (of many!) variations on the basic setup statement that you can use and change to fit your experience:

> Even though I <describe your MPI>, I completely love, accept and forgive myself and anyone else.
>
> Even though I <describe your MPI>, I choose to forgive myself now.
>
> Even though I <describe your MPI>, I accept and forgive myself.
>
> Even though I <describe your MPI>, I allow myself to be the way I am.
>
> Even though I <describe your MPI>, I'm willing to let go.
>
> Even though I <describe your MPI>, I'm willing to hold a new perspective.
>
> Even though I <describe your MPI>, it's over and I'm safe now.
>
> Even though I <describe your MPI>, I choose to release this stress now.

> ## THE CHOICES METHOD
>
> EFT expert Dr. Patricia Carrington's Choices Method is another great option for creating your setup statement. Using her method, you counter what you're feeling with the expression "and I choose to . . ." at the end. For example, if you're feeling frustrated, you could use the setup statement:
>
> "Even though I'm feeling frustrated with how my child is behaving right now, I choose to feel calm and patient and release this frustration now."

Step 4: Choose a Reminder Phrase

The reminder phrase is short—just a few words that describe your issue. After you say your setup statement 3 times while Tapping on the Karate Chop point (see page 17), you will speak your reminder phrase out loud at each of the additional eight points in the Tapping sequence (see page 17). For example, if your setup statement has to do with worry or anxiety about a work deadline, you might tap through each point in the sequence saying, "This anxiety about my deadline . . . this anxiety about my deadline . . . this anxiety about my deadline . . ."

You're repeating the reminder phrase out loud to remind yourself of the issue at each point. This reminder phrase serves to keep your focus on your MPI so you don't get distracted. It also acts as a barometer, helping you determine how focusing on your MPI makes you feel, both physically and emotionally.

Once you get used to Tapping, you can change your reminder phrase as you tap through each point. For example, you might say, "All this anxiety about my work deadline . . . so anxious about this project . . . so much anxiety about this deadline." I will offer this kind of evolving reminder phrase in the Tapping scripts throughout the book. But to start with, feel free to keep it simple and say the same statement at each point.

Step 5: Tap through the Points

Once you have created your setup statement and your reminder phrase, you're ready to start Tapping. You'll start by repeating your setup statement 3 times, while Tapping on the Karate Chop point. You can tap with whichever hand feels most comfortable to you. Tap at a pace and with a force that feel right; you can't get it wrong!

After you've said the setup statement 3 times, you'll move on to Tapping through the eight points in the Tapping sequence, while repeating the reminder phrase. These points are:

- Eyebrow
- Side of eye
- Under eye
- Under nose
- Chin
- Collarbone
- Under arm
- Top of head

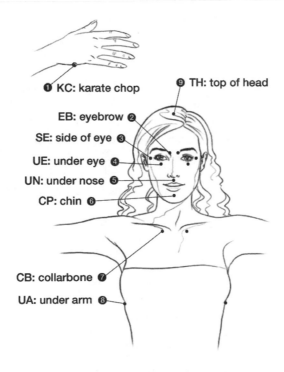

You can tap with either hand, on whichever side of the body feels best to you, because the same meridian channels run down both sides of the body. You can even tap both sides of the body at once if you'd like (it's not necessary, however, as you'll hit the same meridian lines, regardless of which side you tap).

Tap 5 to 7 times at each stop as you work through the sequence. This doesn't have to be an exact count. If it feels right to tap 20 times—or 100—on one point, then do it! The idea is simply to spend enough time at that point to speak your reminder phrase and let it sink in. Don't worry about being perfect—just do what feels right and have the experience.

Step 6: Check In

You've now completed a round of Tapping! First things first: Take a deep breath. Feel your body and notice what's happening. Did you experience a shift of any kind–in your emotions or in your body? How intense does your MPI feel on the 0-to-10 scale now? If your MPI went from an 8 to a 7, that's huge! It means that Tapping is beginning to relieve your stress. It means a shift happened in just a matter of minutes, so keep Tapping. If there's no change, that's fine, too. It's common for people to need more than one round of Tapping to experience relief, especially as they are first becoming familiar with the process.

As you check in with yourself to see if you experienced any shift, ask yourself a few questions:

- What sensations did I experience in my body while Tapping?

- What emotions came up while I was Tapping?

- What "random" thoughts or memories came to mind as I was Tapping?

YAWNING, SIGHING, BURPING & MORE

People often ask if they're doing something wrong, since each time they tap, they begin yawning or experiencing other physical effects. These are all good signs! They're ways that your body is relaxing, moving and releasing energy and letting go. When you tap, make a point of noticing all these ways in which your body responds.

SWITCHING FROM THE "NEGATIVE" TO THE "POSITIVE"

Throughout the book, each Tapping script begins with the "negative," a statement that includes your MPI, and any related challenging emotions and beliefs. Most of the time, I'll end with at least one "positive" round of Tapping, which presents a new way of moving forward.

As a general rule, it's best to get the intensity of the negative down to a 5 out of 10 before moving on to the positive, and then to keep Tapping on the positive until the negative emotional charge has decreased to a 3 or lower.

As you tap, remember to tune in to any shifts you experience in your body and emotions, small or large. Tune in to how your body and your emotional state are shifting. Tune in to new insights and feelings as you tap.

TAPPING TIP: STICK WITH ME . . .

If you find yourself Tapping but not noticing any changes yet, don't be concerned. The process happens differently for everyone. Some people see immediate results, for others it may take a little longer. If you're feeling panicked about getting results for your child, then tap on it! If you feel frustrated or scared that this process won't work for your child, make sure to include those emotions in your Tapping.

To most people, Tapping seems strange at first. It takes a little effort to memorize the points and understand the process. But stick with me through the process and take the time to really learn the basic steps.

Step 7: Test Your Progress

Once the intensity of your MPI has decreased, it's time to test your results. You can do this by refocusing your attention on your MPI. For example, if your MPI was stress around a fight you had with your teenager this morning, you might envision the fight and then check in with yourself to notice how intense that memory now feels. If the memory still feels emotionally charged, continue Tapping through a few more rounds using the same language, and see if you can clear your MPI altogether.

Or you might find that as you think about your argument, instead of feeling angry, you feel sad. That's great! That's an indication that you're getting to the root of your MPI. In that case, you can move on and tap on your sadness, and see where that leads you.

TAPPING PROCESS: QUICK REFERENCE GUIDE

Now that we've been through the Tapping process in detail, here's a quick step-by-step guide for reference:

- To start, close your eyes and take 3 deep breaths. Feel yourself grounded in your body and focused on the present moment. Feel your feet firmly planted on the ground, rooted to the earth. We want to give this process and your body all the attention they deserve, so take a few moments to become present.
- Focus on your MPI and devise a reminder phrase (see page 14).
- Rate the intensity of your MPI on the 0 to 10 SUDS (see page 14), with 10 being the most intensity you can imagine. Take note of this number.
- Craft a setup statement (see page 14).
- Tap on the Karate Chop point (see page 17) while repeating your setup statement 3 times.
- Tap through the eight points in the EFT sequence (see page 17) while saying your reminder phrase out loud. Tap 5 to 7 times at each point, but don't worry about counting or doing it perfectly; it's a forgiving process.
- Once you have finished Tapping the points in the sequence, take a deep breath.
- Again rate the intensity of your MPI using the 0-to-10 scale to check your progress.
- Repeat as necessary to get the relief you desire.
- It can be helpful to write down the shifts you experience in your MPI, as well as your emotions and your body. Remember, shifts in all of these areas mean progress!

GOING WITH THE FLOW

As you continue Tapping, both on your own and with your child, you'll eventually have an experience akin to what we call "peeling the onion." Whatever MPI is being tapped on in any given round is called the "target." As you tap, different layers or aspects of that target will arise. Often you start with one target and then find something else underneath it—a layer!

For example, your child's initial target might be the anxiety he feels about an upcoming test. As you tap on that anxiety, it may shift—and at the same time, he may remember something that someone said to him that makes him feel that he has to get top grades all of the time. That pressure to perform perfectly all of the time may actually be what's holding him back.

These kinds of progressions are good, even when they don't seem to make sense or to be connected in any obvious way. As we'll see in future chapters, for yourself and especially with kids, it's crucial to let the process flow naturally.

RAPID TRANSFORMATION IS POSSIBLE

As you begin to tap, keep in mind that this process can happen a lot more quickly than you might imagine. In my 10+ years of Tapping with hundreds of thousands of people around the world, I've seen countless people of all ages move through multiple layers of an MPI and move the intensity from a 9 or 10 down to a 1 or 0 in anywhere from 5 to 20+ minutes. For others it may take two or 3 sessions, or more. Let the process flow, and trust that transformations can and do happen a lot quicker than you might expect.

THE TAPPING TREE

There are four common types of layers, or Tapping targets, that we will work with throughout this book: *symptoms/side effects*, *emotions*, *events* and *limiting beliefs*.

In order to help you identify these targets in your mind, I'd like to introduce you to a great visual called The Tapping Tree, a concept that was created by my friend and EFT expert Lindsay Kenny. This creative visual shows each target category and how it affects particular targets.

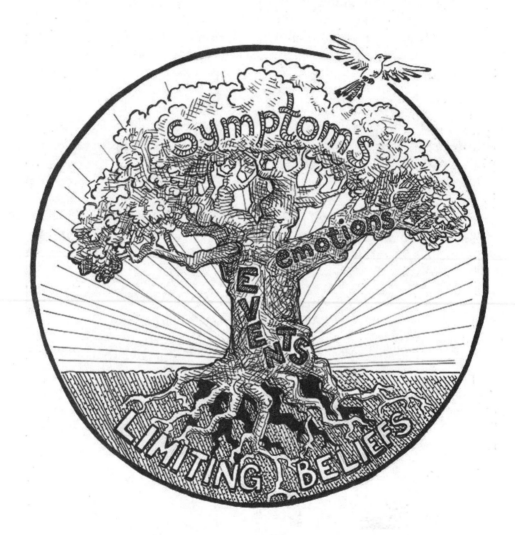

Symptoms/Side Effects (The Leaves): Physical sensations (tingling, heart racing, hot/cold, pain, nausea, etc.), avoidance, procrastination, self-sabotage, disagreements, inability to focus, hyper-activity, bullying, eating issues (picky eater, over-eating, lack of appetite, etc.) and so on.

Emotions (The Branches): Shame, guilt, remorse, rejection, anger, resentment, sadness, depression, powerlessness, fear, anxiety, stress and so on.

Events (The Trunk): Test taking, being bullied, divorce, detached parents, abandonment/betrayal, abuse in any form, excessive discipline/criticism, physical punishment, family fighting/shouting, feeling unsupported or unloved, living with an alcoholic parent or child and so on.

Limiting Beliefs (The Roots): "My child never does well in school," "I'm just not good at taking tests," "There's nothing I can do," "I have ADD/anxiety disorder/etc.," "I hate school," "He/she/I am a bad/stupid/etc. student/child" and so on.

Throughout the rest of the book, we'll skip around to various points in The Tapping Tree—Tapping on the symptoms/side effects, emotions, traumatic events, and underlying beliefs alike. You may find that when you tap on one part of the tree, such as test anxiety, for example, another part of the tree, such as a headache, goes away or shifts in some way. The tree isn't necessarily a top-down or bottom-up system, since all parts feed each other and can be interrelated, but it's a useful visual to help you recognize the different aspects of an issue.

ACCESSING A WIDER RANGE OF EMOTIONS

Sometimes it's easy to get stuck on the emotions we're most familiar with. For example, many of us end up Tapping on stress and feelings of anxiety and frustration, which are easy to recognize. But accessing a broader emotional vocabulary can help bring more specificity to Tapping. Here are some key emotions many of us experience. Use this list to further connect with what's going on for you.

Alienation	Envy	Hysteria
Ambivalence	Fear	Insecurity
Anger	Frustration	Loathing
Anxiety	Fury	Loneliness

Bitterness	Grief	Paranoia
Boredom	Grouchiness	Pity
Contempt	Guilt	Rage
Depression	Hatred	Regret
Despair	Homesickness	Remorse
Disgust	Hope	Resentment
Distress	Horror	Shame
Doubt	Hostility	Suffering
Dread	Humiliation	Worry
Embarrassment	Hunger	

RELIEF WHEN YOU NEED IT

One of the amazing benefits of EFT is how quickly it can produce real, long-lasting stress relief for people of all ages. Sometimes you or your child may tap on an issue and get immediate and lasting relief. At other times it may take longer. As we've seen, our brains are hardwired to resist change of all kinds. That hardwired resistance may even have made your brain adept at avoiding the emotions it doesn't want to face. From one person to another and from one issue to the next, the process will vary. What's important is to keep tapping whenever you can and for whatever period of time you can—even if it's just the 60 seconds before taking an exam.

TAPPING EXERCISE (OPTIONAL): CREATING YOUR OWN TAPPING TREE

Some people find it helpful to create their own Tapping tree. To download a copy of The Tapping Tree exercise, visit https://www.thetappingsolution.com/tree/.

WHEN SHOULD YOU TAP?

Whether you're Tapping for yourself or with your child, I recommend Tapping whenever there's stress, discomfort (physical, mental or emotional), or distress of any kind.

There's no wrong time to tap, and it's impossible to tap too much.

Some people find it helpful to make a habit of always Tapping at a certain time of day, like first thing in the morning, after school, or in the evenings before bed. If there's a time of day when it's easier to take a few minutes of quiet time to tap, do that. If it's best to pick a different time each day, do that. I've known many people who regularly tap in class or at the office, in bathroom stalls, on airplanes, and when they're stopped at red lights.

You can also tap when you're in a challenging situation, like when you're having a difficult phone conversation, or struggling to focus while studying or working. The simple act of Tapping will help to calm your mind and body. You can then do more focused Tapping on releasing any resulting emotions or experiences later. Whenever you or your child needs relief of any kind, just start Tapping!

AREN'T EMOTIONS A *GOOD* THING? WHY DO WE TAP ON RELEASING THEM?

People sometimes ask me why we focus on releasing emotions when we're Tapping. Aren't emotions a good thing?

Yes, they absolutely are!

Our goal with Tapping is never to stop feeling our emotions. Instead, Tapping helps us to acknowledge how we're feeling, and then feel them *more* fully. When we can do that, our emotions naturally progress. For instance, if you tap on anger, that anger may then turn into sadness, which then becomes compassion.

As a result of this emotional processing and release, which often happens faster with Tapping, we become more present in the moment. That presence then supports healthier relationships with ourselves and with our children.

Let's look at how that might play out in everyday life:

Have you ever had the same fight with the same person over and over again? For instance, maybe you and your high-school-aged child get in a fight, or at least have a difficult discussion, around homework most nights. As soon as the topic is raised, you both tense, and before long, you're replaying the same fight you've had dozens, if not hundreds, of times. It's incredibly frustrating!

With Tapping, you can put an end to that pattern.

Using that same example, let's say one night you decide to tap on that fight you just had with your child around homework. While Tapping, you realize that you're worried that your child will make the same mistake you made by not taking school seriously enough and then paying the price for it later. While Tapping through your worry, you realize that you've been holding onto regret and sadness about how ostracized and unsupported you felt when you were in school. After about 10 minutes of Tapping, you feel relaxed and relieved, like a huge burden has been lifted.

The next night, when the topic of homework arises, you're able to remain calm. As a result, you and your child have an honest, open discussion about why you've been having the same fight for so long. Suddenly, the pattern has been interrupted and you and your child begin finding new ways of communicating about homework. Amazing!

That's the power of Tapping. It allows you to feel your emotions more fully, not less, so that you can be present in what's happening now, rather than being distracted by past, repressed emotion.

Before we look at how to use Tapping to transform your experience around parenting, let's do a few quick rounds of Tapping.

Tapping Exercise: **Releasing Anxiety**

Since you're reading this book, I'm guessing that you're seeking results of some kind. Often at the start of a process like this, people feel anxious about getting results immediately, especially when the results they're wanting are for their child. That impatience creates stress, which, as we've seen, keeps you stuck in negative patterns. Let's do a few quick Tapping rounds to lower that stress.

Begin by focusing on your impatience around getting results now. Say out loud, "I'm so frustrated that this problem isn't improving fast enough" (or some other similar phrase). How intense does that feel on a scale of 0 to 10? Give it a number.

We'll begin by Tapping 3 times on the Karate Chop point:

Karate Chop *(Repeat 3 times)*: Even though I need results from Tapping now, especially for my child, I love myself and accept how I feel.

Eyebrow: I need results now

Side of Eye: I can't wait

Under Eye: I don't have that kind of time

Under Nose: I need to help my child now

Under Mouth: So much pressure

Collarbone: So much stress

Under Arm: All this anxiety

Top of Head: I need results now

Eyebrow: Feeling so impatient

Side of Eye: So stressed out

Under Eye: This stress isn't helping me

Under Nose: This stress is holding me back

Under Mouth: The sooner I shed this stress, the sooner I can help my child

Collarbone: Releasing this stress now

Under Arm: Letting go of this impatience

Top of Head: Releasing it from every cell in my body now

Eyebrow: It's safe to feel calm

Side of Eye: It's safe to feel patient

Under Eye: The calmer I am, the more I can help my child

Under Nose: Allowing myself to feel calm and patient now

Under Mouth: Allowing myself to feel quiet and calm now

Collarbone: Allowing myself to relax into this process

Under Arm: Allowing myself to feel calm and relaxed now

Top of Head: Allowing myself to feel calm and relaxed now

Take a deep breath. Check back in on the intensity of the stress and impatience you're feeling around getting immediate Tapping results. Give it a number on a scale of 0 to 10. Keep Tapping until you get the relief you desire.

In the next chapter, we'll focus on one of the biggest blocks that parents experience—overwhelm.

Chapter 3

Releasing Parental Overwhelm

It wasn't long ago that parents had little information about what "good" parenting looked like. Parents had one, maybe two, parenting books that were considered credible. Today we face the opposite problem. From conscious parenting to authoritative parenting, attachment parenting and more, we're bombarded with drastically different and increasingly detailed definitions of what a "good" parent looks like.

As helpful as this information can sometimes be, it often creates the impression that our own parenting is under scrutiny. We wonder, "Am I doing the 'right' things to support my child's academic, social and emotional development? Am I giving them too much access to technology, or not enough? Involving them in too many extracurricular activities, or too few? And in the midst of our busy days, how can I best respond to their ever-changing behavior, habits and attitude?"

The list of important, challenging questions parents face each day is overwhelming, and even more so for single parents and parents of children with developmental delays. As tempting as it is to rush in and "fix" our parenting, and by extension our children, research suggests that the best place to start is by releasing our own stress.

A study of 1,037 parents published by the American Psychological Association (APA) found that while 69% of parents said that their stress has little to no effect on their children, 91% of children reported knowing when a parent was stressed by observing behaviors like yelling, arguing and complaining. In addition, the kids who reported being aware of their parents' stress were generally more likely to feel sad, worried and frustrated. They were also significantly more likely to exhibit stress symptoms themselves.[1]

My intention in sharing these findings is not to cause you additional worry. Whatever you do, don't stress about your stress! The fact is, parenting is stressful. It's a huge responsibility, and any stress you feel is a reflection of how deeply you care. That's a wonderful thing!

I'm sharing these research findings for two reasons:

1) so that you know you're not alone; and

2) so that you'll take a little bit of time in these next few chapters to focus on relieving your own stress before Tapping with your children.

This chapter and the four that follow it are intended to give you some well-earned relief. They're a chance to shed some stress, as well as other emotions, and feel a bit better. I hope you'll stick with me, even if your primary motivation for reading this book is to use Tapping with your kids.

Once your own batteries have been recharged, you'll be in a calmer, quieter place, which is when Tapping with your kids is likely to feel easier and more productive. It's like the airplane instructions that tell you to put your oxygen mask on yourself first, before putting one on your child. Once you've done your own Tapping, you're more protected from the stress of feeling overwhelmed. At that point you're better equipped to support your child.

In this chapter we'll begin by looking at some of the limiting beliefs that may be fueling the feelings of overwhelm that so many of us experience.

> ### *TAPPING TIP*: RELEASING LIMITING BELIEFS
>
> Beliefs are the foundation of our worlds. They shape the way we see, feel and experience our lives. That's why limiting beliefs often feel like "the truth."
>
> Beliefs can be the cumulative result of lessons we learned as children and perhaps again later in life. There may even be 1,000 different things that we've heard, seen or done that created a single belief. Fortunately, with Tapping we don't have to clear all 1,000 events to get relief, but we may need to dig deeper to find the handful of memories or events that together act as the foundation for that belief.
>
> That's also why some beliefs take longer to release. If you find yourself Tapping on the same belief(s) repeatedly, don't be discouraged. That's normal. The biggest transformations often happen when we let go of limiting beliefs that no longer serve us, so keep Tapping on them, and remember to appreciate every bit of progress you make along the way.

LIMITING BELIEF #1: "I DON'T HAVE TIME FOR MYSELF"

It was a chilly evening in December several years ago when Dr. Lori Leyden of the Tapping Solution Foundation first sat down with a group of adults, a Tapping group intended to resolve the stress they were all feeling as parents. After introducing herself, Lori asked each attendee to share why they had come and what was going on in their lives.

One after another, Lori listened as parents expressed their feeling that they *couldn't* take a break. Instead of pausing to appreciate how much they were handling every day, they were overcome with anxiety at the thought of taking time out to release the feelings of overwhelm they were shouldering.

Like Lori, I have often heard these same refrains from parents:

"I don't have time to take a break!"

"I'm always there for my family. I don't have time for myself."

"Someone always needs something. I don't get time for me."

Although I haven't been doing this parenting job for very long, I get it. After years of watching friends and family care for their kids, I've gotten a sense of how endless the job of parenting can seem. There's so much to do, so much to pay attention to and take care of, that parents feel incredible pressure to prioritize their kids over themselves. Our children are precious beyond words. How could we not give our all to care for them?

As we've seen, though, when stress becomes chronic, it has increasingly negative effects on our children's and our own health and well-being. James Clear, a writer and motivational speaker, explains the effects of cumulative stress this way:

"Imagine that your health and energy are a bucket of water.

In your day-to-day life, there are things that fill your bucket up. These are inputs like sleep, nutrition, meditation, stretching, laughter and other forms of recovery.

There are also forces that drain the water from your bucket. These are outputs like lifting weights or running, stress from work or school, relationship problems or other forms of stress and anxiety.

The forces that drain your bucket aren't all negative, of course. To live a productive life, it is important to have some things flowing out of your bucket. Working hard in the gym, at school or at the office allows you to produce something of value. But even positive outputs are still *outputs* and they drain your energy accordingly.

These outputs are cumulative. Even a little leak can result in significant water loss over time."[2]

When it comes to parenting, maintaining a healthy balance gets trickier, in part because our children fill and empty our buckets faster and in more extreme ways than nearly anything else in our lives.

At one moment, they're waking you up at 3 AM *again* (draining your bucket), only to drift back off to sleep with a look so peaceful, your heart swells with love and gratitude (filling your bucket). And just when you're sure they'll never help around the house (draining your bucket), you arrive home one evening to find the dinner prepared and their homework done (filling your bucket).

Since you can't control how and when these moments will happen, the key to maintaining a positive equilibrium from one day to the next is to take time to fill your own bucket. According to research, though, even parents who believe that stress relief needs to be high on their priority list aren't taking time to lower their stress. That same study published by the American Psychological Association found that while 69% of parents believe that managing their stress is important, only 32% feel they are doing an excellent or very good job of doing that.[3]

What's going on here? Why aren't parents taking time to relieve their own stress?

Although we may tell ourselves, "I don't have time for myself," my sense is that being crunched for time is only part of the issue. Just as significant a contributing factor is how much value our culture places on doing and achieving over feeling and being. You may notice this in the way you spend and value your own time.

For example, at the end of a long and busy day, instead of viewing your exhaustion as a reason to slow down, you may praise yourself for being productive. "I'm exhausted, but I got a lot done today," you might say. You then set an intention to be equally or more productive tomorrow. The cycle goes on and on. No matter how much you accomplish, you have a persistent, nagging feeling that you need to do more.

Even when you know you need a break, you may feel uncomfortable about taking time for the kind of self-care that "fills your bucket." When faced with an opportunity, instead of taking time for yourself, you squeeze in more things for your kids, your family, your employer—anyone and everyone *except* yourself!

By always expecting yourself to do and give more, however, you allow the leaks in your health and wellness buckets to turn into major losses—of patience, energy, resilience, health and well-being. Since you and your kids deserve the best of you, let's take a few minutes now to do some Tapping on releasing any discomfort you feel about taking time for yourself.

Tapping Exercise: I Don't Have Time for Myself

First ask yourself how true the statement "I don't have time for myself" feels on a scale of 0 to 10. You can say it in your head or speak it out loud. Take note of that number and also notice what you feel in your body as you repeat that statement. Is there any anxiety or stress? What other thoughts come to mind when you say that statement? Notice them, bring them forward into your consciousness, and we'll start Tapping.

Take 3 deep breaths, allowing yourself to feel grounded in your body. We'll begin by Tapping 3 times on the Karate Chop point:

Karate Chop *(Repeat 3 times)*: Even though I have this belief that I don't have time for myself, I deeply and completely love and accept myself.

Eyebrow: I can't take time for myself

Side of Eye: There's so much to do

Under Eye: I can't take time for myself

Under Nose: I don't *have* that kind of time!

Under Mouth: There's so much I need to get done

Collarbone: And so much my kids need from me

Under Arm: I don't have time for myself

Top of Head: I *can't* take time for myself

Eyebrow: All this stress around taking time for myself

Side of Eye: I need to be there for my kids

Under Eye: And for my family and friends

Under Nose: There's so much to do

Under Mouth: I don't have time to give to myself

Collarbone: This stress isn't good for me, though

Under Arm: It exhausts me

Top of Head: This stress depletes me

Eyebrow: What if taking time to tap helped me feel better?

Side of Eye: What if a few minutes of Tapping gave me more energy and patience to give to my children?

Under Eye: I can take a few minutes for myself

Under Nose: I can release this discomfort around taking time for myself

Under Mouth: And tap whenever I feel stressed out

Collarbone: It's safe to take time for myself

Under Arm: Releasing all of this stress now

Top of Head: Allowing myself to feel calm and relaxed now

Take a deep breath, and check in with yourself. How true does the statement "I don't have time for myself" feel now, on a scale of 0 to 10? You can say it in your head or speak it out loud. What else came up as we were doing that Tapping? What other ideas/thoughts/emotions? Perhaps you thought of your mother, who always ran the "perfect ship." Pay attention to other things that come up and, if it's helpful, write them down. These are all clues to what's really going on, and they will point you toward how to get the best relief.

You can either tap further on this issue (the couple of rounds here are just to get you started; make sure to do as much as you need), or you can move on to other issues that might have come up.

LIMITING BELIEF #2: "THERE'S NEVER ENOUGH TIME!"

The fact is there *are* only so many hours in a day. When you're juggling family, home, school, work, finances, homework, extra-curricular activities and more, time becomes incredibly precious. While you may yearn for more quality time, family time and down time, those things take time you don't have. You do everything possible to "make" time, but still end most days asking yourself, *where did the time go?*

Caught in this cycle of doing more and more, without realizing it, you may ratchet up your expectations of what you *should* be able to accomplish during a given day or week. As a result, no matter how much you're doing, it continues to feel like there's never enough time. By taking a moment to pause and appreciate all that you are doing, you can begin to create a new relationship with time. Once you've shed stress around never having enough time, you can become more present in the time that you do have.

Tapping Exercise: There's Never Enough Time

Let's take a moment now to tap on the belief that there's never enough time. To begin, focus on the statement, "There's never enough time." You can say it in your head or out loud. How true does that statement feel on a scale of 0 to 10?

Notice what you feel in your body as you say that statement. Do you experience any tightness, clenching, pain or discomfort in your body? What else comes up for you when you think about not having enough time? Do you think of certain people, or find yourself thinking about a certain part of your life? Does an old memory come up? Notice what you feel.

Take 3 deep breaths. We'll start by Tapping 3 times on the Karate Chop point.

Karate Chop *(Repeat 3 times)*: Even though I have this belief that there's never enough time, I deeply and completely love and accept myself.

Eyebrow: There's never enough time

Side of Eye: It's the truth

Under Eye: There's never enough time

Under Nose: There are always more things to do

Under Mouth: There's never enough time

Collarbone: It's a fact

Under Arm: I'd love more quality time with my family

Top of Head: More quiet time with my kids

Eyebrow: But there's never enough time

Side of Eye: I have so much to do

Under Eye: There's so much that HAS to get done

Under Nose: I try to "make" time for other things

Under Mouth: But still, there's never enough time

Collarbone: It's stressful

Under Arm: What if my stress around time is the real issue here?

Top of Head: What if I could trust that there is enough time?

Eyebrow: Releasing this belief that there's never enough time

Side of Eye: I'm doing a lot already!

Under Eye: It's safe to appreciate all that I'm already doing

Under Nose: It's safe to release this stress around time now

Under Mouth: I can trust that there is enough time

Collarbone: I can appreciate everything that I'm already doing

Under Arm: Allowing myself to trust that there *is* enough time

Top of Head: Allowing myself to feel calm and present in this moment now

Take 3 deep breaths. How true does the belief, "There's never enough time" feel now? Give it a number on a scale of 0 to 10.

As before, pay attention to what comes up as you're Tapping—that will help you delve deeper and peel that onion.

"I can't tap right now. I only have a minute."

That's fine! If you've got a minute to spare while your kids are getting in the bath or putting on their shoes, sometimes that's all you need. Do a round or two while you're waiting. If you have a favorite Tapping point (lots of people get fast relief from the collarbone point, for example), feel free to use that minute, or even just a few seconds, to tap on that one point.

LIMITING BELIEF #3: "I'M TOO TIRED"

Having spent so many years going and doing, it's no wonder we hear ourselves saying, "I'm too tired" so often! Even a good night's sleep often doesn't restore our energy. The question is, then, are we really too tired, or are we suffering from the effects of chronic stress?

As Dr. Christiane Northrup, MD, shares in her book *Goddesses Never Age*, decreased energy is not an inevitable result of the aging process:

> "In truth, what we call 'aging' is chronic deterioration as you move through time. While its accumulative effects typically show up later, this kind of aging actually begins in your 20s when you start sitting all day. And then it gets progressively worse the older you get.
>
> This deterioration is not inevitable! You have the power to change your experience, no matter what 'runs in your family' or what you've been told. If deterioration is essentially optional, then you can write a new script, follow a new path. You can actually become biologically younger this year than you were last year. It all starts with your beliefs. And the behavior that follows."[4]

The good news is when we lower stress, we allow the body to restore itself and regain energy. In doing so, we can prevent, and perhaps even reverse, any deterioration that has taken place.

Tapping Exercise: I'm Too Tired

Now that we've done some Tapping on creating a positive belief around having the time you need, let's make some space for the possibility that you have all of the energy you need as well.

To begin, say out loud, "I'm too tired." How true does that statement feel on a scale of 0 to 10? Give it a number.

Also notice what you feel in your body as you say that statement either in your head or out loud. What gives you energy and what seems to take it away? When did you start feeling too tired? Notice what comes up.

Take 3 deep breaths. We'll start by tapping 3 times on the Karate Chop point.

Karate Chop (*Repeat 3 times*): Even though I'm often too tired to do everything I need and want to do, I deeply and completely love and accept myself.

Eyebrow: I'm too tired

Side of Eye: I don't have the energy I need

Under Eye: So tired

Under Nose: I don't have the energy I used to have

Under Mouth: I'm too tired

Collarbone: So much to do

Under Arm: So much to think about

Top of Head: So much to plan

Eyebrow: I'm too tired

Side of Eye: Don't have the energy I used to

Under Eye: I'm too tired

Under Nose: It's a part of getting older

Under Mouth: It's a part of being a parent

Collarbone: I don't like feeling so tired

Under Arm: I'm tired of feeling too tired

Top of Head: Maybe it's my stress that's exhausting me

Eyebrow: I'm sick of this stress

Side of Eye: I can let go of my stress

Under Eye: Releasing my stress and fatigue now

Under Nose: Without this stress, I can get my energy back!

Under Mouth: Releasing this belief that I'm too tired now

Collarbone: I can feel energized again

Under Arm: I can let go of this stress and exhaustion

Top of Head: And allow myself to feel energized now

Take 3 deep breaths, and check in with yourself again. On a scale of 0 to 10, how true does the belief "I'm too tired" feel now? Keep Tapping until you get the relief you desire.

NEGOTIATING THE "PERFECT PARENT" SYNDROME

Another way we are all constantly confronted with the stress of having to be the best possible parent is through social media. Have you ever logged onto Facebook or Instagram to see picture after picture of families arguing on holidays, kids having meltdowns at birthday parties, and siblings fighting on vacation? Or seen pictures of parents looking fed up with the constant cleaning, scheduling, and refereeing required during their latest family event?

Of course not! Because most of what people post on social media paints quite a different picture from reality. But in this age of social media, where more of our lives are being broadcast online at the touch of a button, our experience of parenting is often being shaped by what is shared online by others and our interpretations of these images.

In the past couple of chapters we've looked at several internal issues around parenting. Now let's see how all of this plays out in the external world.

FACEBOOK'S FAIRY TALES

As children, most of us celebrated our birthdays with a handful of friends, some form of cake, balloons and maybe a piñata. Today, children's birthday parties have become so elaborate that there's a backlash in mainstream media, parenting blogs and social media about returning to the simpler celebrations we knew as children.

At the center of that backlash, though, it's hard to ignore the stream of idyllic party pictures on social media. Even if we yearn to simplify, we can't help but wonder how our children would experience a simpler celebration. Will they feel slighted? Will the people we don't invite, in order to keep the gathering small and simple, be upset at us—or worse, our children?

Social media and birthday parties are, of course, just two of the many examples of how the external world can intimately affect our experience of parenting. In addition to worrying about our kids, we too, may feel pressured to conform to the "perfect" images that we see on social media of families looking happy, healthy and engaged. And let's be honest here—it can be fun posting a picture and getting tons of positive comments and likes. And there's absolutely nothing wrong with that! By sharing important parts of our lives with people we care about, we feel more supported. That's a great thing!

At the same time though, social media can be a source of pressure and stress. After all, if on the afternoon of a holiday riddled by tantrums and fights in your house you log onto social media and see happy, smiling photos of friends and their families celebrating that same holiday, you may secretly wonder what went "wrong" in your house.

This habit of comparing ourselves to others isn't new, of course, but it is happening on a larger and more frequent scale, thanks to the technology at our fingertips. The pressure that parents are feeling as a result of social media was discussed in an October 2015 cover article in *Time* magazine on parenting in the digital age. The article described what we, as parents, see online as "an impossibly pristine, accomplished version of their family lives on the web." The article went on to add:

> "In scores of interviews for this article, just the mention of social media elicited groans and sighs from young parents who are barraged by hand-made birthday invitations and color-coded clothespin chore charts on Pinterest. They debate whether Facebook or Instagram is 'the hardest,' whether it's the images of the home-cooked organic feast or the just-cleaned house.
>
> It helps only a little to know that people are being highly selective about what they share. 'Someone will put out there, "Oh, I just braided my child's hair." But you just yelled at them like 50 times to sit down,' says 30-year-old B. Marcell Williams, a mother of four."[5]

Have you ever felt pressured by social media or some other community to be the "perfect parent" or to host the "perfect" children's event? If so, has that pressure affected the way you see yourself as a parent, and how you interact with your partner, children and friends?

"Living a meaningful life is not a popularity contest. If what you're saying is always getting applause, you're probably not yet doing the right stuff."
— Marianne Williamson at the 2015 Parliament of the World's Religions

To begin, let's do a simple but powerful Tapping exercise around generating more awareness of where stress may be coming from when it comes to social media.

EXERCISE: NOTICING STRESS PATTERNS AROUND SOCIAL MEDIA

Open one of your preferred social media outlets, whether it's Facebook, Pinterest, Instagram or something else, and look through your feed. When you see "perfect" pictures of other parents, families and their children, how do you feel?

Pause when you come upon a photo or video that creates any kind of negative reaction—whether it's judgment, jealousy, irritation, even hesitation.

Begin Tapping as you look at the photo or video that's causing a reaction. As you're Tapping, ask yourself questions like:

- What do I feel in my body when I look at this?
- What's the main emotion I feel when I look at this?
- What am I telling myself when I look at this?

The answers to these questions are your Tapping targets.

For instance, if you're looking at a photo and telling yourself that you're not good enough, or that you're not doing enough for your family, tap on that belief. Notice any emotions, from shame to guilt, anxiety and more, that come up. Keep Tapping until you can look at that same image and feel less of an emotional charge.

To further your awareness of the causes of "good" versus "bad" stress in your life, I encourage you to do this same exercise around photos, videos, memories and events that elicit a positive reaction. It's a great opportunity to tap in to positive energy, and notice more sources of "good" stress.

LIMITING BELIEF #4: GIVING YOUR "BEST EVER!" GIFT

When we see "perfect party" pictures, naturally we want to give that same experience to our children. However, if by the day of the party your home is rife with fighting, money is tight, and you feel like you're just holding on until the party is over, you're experiencing "bad" stress.

Keep in mind, my intention here is not to judge anyone—myself included!—but to point out that there's often a discrepancy between real life experiences and how they appear to others, both online and offline. What if instead of focusing on the "perfect party/holiday/weekend," we focused on being the best versions of ourselves?

The fact is, even when your children don't act like it, the best and most important gift you can give them is always a happy, healthy YOU. By making your own health and happiness your top priority, you're giving them your greatest gift—your complete presence.

As we discussed earlier in this chapter, taking care of yourself first is so important to your children. Think about it for a moment.

If you factored your health and well-being into more of your parenting decisions, would you make the same decisions you made in the past? If taking time for Tapping, sleep, exercise, hobbies, etc. were higher priorities, would your home and family life be different?

Let's take a look at a common limiting belief that prevents us from making our own health and well-being a higher priority in how we live and parent.

EXERCISE: WHO COMES FIRST? CONFLICTING BELIEFS ABOUT PARENTING

Have you ever heard yourself say something like, *I was exhausted, but the kids loved it, so I guess it was worth it?*

There are times, of course, when going above and beyond is necessary and important in helping our children grow and thrive. However, making a regular habit of sacrificing our needs on behalf of our children causes us to take on beliefs like:

Parenting is about self-sacrifice.

It's all about my kids. I don't count.

My kids always come first.

My kids' happiness is more important than my own.

While these beliefs may contain some truth, they don't serve us, or our kids, when they're seen as the whole truth. As a result of beliefs like these, we experience more stress and less joy. In that stressed-out state, as we've seen, we no longer bring our best selves to our parenting.

Take a moment now to think back on a time when you felt like you had to sacrifice yourself in some way on behalf of your children; or a time when you put your kids' happiness in front of your own.

Begin Tapping through the points as you paint the picture in your mind of what was happening and how you felt.

When you think of that time, whether it was a holiday celebration, science project or soccer season, on a scale of 0 to 10, how true does the statement *I had to sacrifice my needs for my kids* feel?

Noticing any emotions you feel when you think of it, continue Tapping through the points until that belief doesn't feel as true.

Next, as you're Tapping through the points, imagine a different version of that event where you take a few minutes to do some Tapping, make sure to get more sleep, exercise, and so on.

This may mean setting firmer boundaries with yourself, your family, and your time. As you envision this new version of the event, picture yourself setting those boundaries.

CUPCAKES ARE DELICIOUS. PERIOD.

During the many years before social pressures begin to dominate their behavior and moods, children know what we, as parents, often forget. They know that cupcakes are delicious, whether they're store-bought, homemade, organic or custom decorated. They know that going to the park can be just as exciting as seeing the newest movie or doing the "perfect" art project. They know that great music feels good, mac and cheese is always yummy and riding a bike rarely disappoints.

What children know that we often forget is that joy is always available. They don't wait until they've cleaned their room to enjoy themselves; they play while they clean, invent games while they eat and sing as they draw, write and color. They don't limit how much or how often they experience joy. Instead, they seize every opportunity to feel it.

In other words, joy happens when they, and we, *choose* to feel it.

As parents, we're often so busy managing logistics, relationships, finances, as well as external pressure to be/act/look certain ways, that joy gets pushed aside. Unfortunately, it's a habit that quickly becomes a vicious cycle, since less joy leads to more stress, which leads to less joy, and so on.

Although we likely can't become childlike again (though there's no harm in trying!), we can allow ourselves to feel more joy more often. In order to do that, we need to begin factoring ourselves—our health, well-being, happiness and yes, joy and laughter—into the equation. If a huge party or celebration is causing more stress than joy, perhaps it's time to consider what you're really giving your children. Are you giving them a truly happy celebration or a household riddled by stress and conflict?

I'm asking you to take your commitment to taking time for yourself to a new level. I'm asking you to consider how parenting can be less about self-sacrifice, and (a lot) more about giving your best self. Will every day be easy, simple and filled with authentic joy? Probably not, but by making a point of injecting more of what lights you up into your daily life and parenting, your experience around parenting *will* change forever.

Next we'll look at how to use Tapping to address another common stressor in parenting—worrying.

Chapter 4

Quieting Worry

"My life has been filled with calamities, some of which actually happened."
– MARK TWAIN

As parents, worry is such an inherent part of our lives that it can seem to be part of our jobs. From birth, or even before, we worry about our children—will they be healthy and happy? Will they be safe? Will they do well in school, make friends, and be prepared for adulthood?

In this chapter, we'll explore the different kinds of worrying that parents experience. We'll also look at how to use Tapping to quiet worrying and increase feelings of safety.

HEALTHY WORRYING VS. "CATASTROPHIZING"

Have you ever heard that some stress is good for you? Studies show that the right amounts of stress can help you to be happier, healthier and more productive. The same can be true of worry. While excessive worrying puts undue stress on you and your child, some worrying can help you successfully anticipate and navigate the different situations we're likely to face as parents.

For example, worrying about your child's new group of friends could prompt you to spend more time getting to know them. That familiarity may give you peace of mind, and/or a clearer picture of how your child's new friends may be influencing him or her. At that point you can take any necessary action.

That's just one example of how worry could be helpful. The challenge with worrying, of course, is figuring out how to turn it into a tool for discovery and growth. That can be tricky when you're a parent, since constructive worry is a slippery slope and can easily turn into something that hurts instead of helps. One indication that worrying is becoming excessive is when it resembles what Brené Brown calls "catastrophizing." She explains how it impacts us this way:

> "Worrying about things that haven't happened doesn't protect us from pain… Instead, catastrophizing, as I call it, squanders the one thing we all want more of in life. We simply cannot know joy without embracing vulnerability—and the way to do that is to focus on *gratitude*, not fear."–Brené Brown[1]

In addition to robbing you of the chance to experience joy, catastrophizing may also cause your kids to feel more anxious than they would otherwise.

Sensing that you don't feel safe in the world, kids naturally assume that they are unsafe also. Rather than keeping them safer, catastrophizing then decreases children's sense of safety.

OVERCOMING CATASTROPHIZING

Kindergarten had been on Wendy's mind for well over a year. The months had passed quickly, and now Ben, her oldest son, would be attending his first day in less than a week. The closer his first day got, the faster Wendy's worries multiplied. Would he be nurtured? Would he feel lost in a much larger school? Most of all, would he be safe?

Ben had loved preschool, and Wendy knew that he was ready for elementary school. However, it had only been nine months since Wendy and her family had moved to a new part of the country. While Ben had handled the many major changes involved in their move incredibly well, kindergarten would be his second new school within the calendar year. Wendy worried that it might be too much for any 5-year-old.

A regular "tapper," Wendy had already done some Tapping on her worries about Ben attending kindergarten. While Tapping had calmed her each time, her worry thoughts always seemed to return. Now that the official start of kindergarten was only days away, she was concerned that Ben would pick up on her anxiety, which in turn might make him nervous.

Determined to stop her worrying for good, Wendy sat down one morning to begin Tapping. After taking a few calming breaths, she realized that her endless worrying didn't make sense. After all, she had taken the school tour, attended registration and orientation meetings, and talked with several other parents whose children already attended that same school. She'd received extremely positive feedback from everyone. Why couldn't she shake this worried feeling?

Realizing this, Wendy decided *not* to tap on her worry, as she had previously. Instead, Wendy tapped through the points while asking herself why she was so scared about Ben attending kindergarten. Due to its relaxing effect on the brain and body, Tapping is also a great tool for self-discovery.

After several rounds of Tapping while asking herself this question, Wendy had an epiphany. She realized that her own childhood experiences with public schools were distorting her perception of Ben's new school.

From a young age, Wendy had seen public schools as dangerous places. As a child growing up in New York City, Wendy and her siblings, all of whom had attended private schools, had been told to stay away from public schools. In those years, the city's crime rates were at all-time highs, and gunfights sometimes broke out in the city's public school parking lots.

To add to Wendy's fears, the shootings that had taken place at Sandy Hook Elementary School (2012), and others around the country more recently, had validated her belief that public schools are unsafe. The thought of Ben being in that kind of danger was petrifying.

As Wendy tapped through her fear that morning, she began to cry. As she continued Tapping on releasing her fear, she felt her entire body relax. Out of the blue, she then envisioned an enormous iridescent bubble protecting Ben's new elementary school. The image felt soothing, so she tapped for a few minutes while holding that image in her mind. By the end of her Tapping that morning, for the first time ever, Wendy felt peaceful when she thought about Ben attending kindergarten.

For the next several days, Wendy continued to tap while imagining that same protective bubble around Ben's new school. As a result of her Tapping, Wendy felt genuinely excited and grateful on Ben's first day.

Ben has since thrived in kindergarten, learning and making new friends with minimal stress or worry.

Have you ever noticed yourself turning worries into imagined catastrophes? No matter how many positive real-world experiences you have, your imagined catastrophes seem almost as real as what's actually happening. That's another example of the brain's negativity bias, which highlights danger over safety, even when your fears are based in your imagination.

By identifying the root cause of her fear and then using Tapping to release it, Wendy was able to increase her own feelings of safety, allowing her to contribute to Ben's excitement about starting kindergarten.

Takeaways for Overcoming Catastrophizing

- If Tapping on your fear or catastrophizing thoughts doesn't provide true relief, use Tapping as a discovery tool. Tap through the points while asking yourself questions like, "What's this fear really about?" and "Why can't I let go of these fears?"

- As Wendy noticed in herself, catastrophizing often has more to do with our own past experiences than those of our children. Pay attention to what events, memories, physical sensations and emotions come up for you when you find yourself spiraling into catastrophizing.

• Once you've released the charge of what was causing your catastrophizing, don't hesitate to use visualization as a way of Tapping in the positive.

Tapping Exercise: Quieting Catastrophizing

When you notice yourself turning regular worry thoughts into catastrophes, the first thing to do is pause and notice that your brain has been hijacked by an *imaginary* catastrophe. Rather than staying stuck in it, you can then do some Tapping to release it. Let's do that now.

Note: If the catastrophe you're dwelling on is related to a past event that you're afraid will recur, turn to the "Releasing Worries That Are Tied to the Past" section later in this chapter.

To begin, take 3 deep breaths. Notice how intense your imagined catastrophe feels on a scale of 0 to 10 and give it a number.

Also notice what you feel in your body as you focus on your catastrophizing fears. What sensations do you feel in your body? Do certain events come to mind? What emotions do you feel?

We'll begin by Tapping 3 times on the Karate Chop point:

Karate Chop *(Repeat 3 times)*: Even though my brain is being hijacked by this scary story of what could happen, I love myself and accept how I feel.

Eyebrow: This imaginary catastrophe

Side of Eye: It feels so real

Under Eye: This scary story

Under Nose: It's hijacking my brain

Under Mouth: It seems so real

Collarbone: It seems like something that could really happen

Under Arm: So scary to think about

Top of Head: It feels like it could really happen

Eyebrow: This scary story

Side of Eye: It's hijacking my brain

Under Eye: It's just a story, though

Under Nose: It's not really happening

Under Mouth: I'm imagining it

Collarbone: And I don't have to believe it

Under Arm: It's just a story

Top of Head: It's not actually happening

Eyebrow: It's safe to release this story

Side of Eye: I don't need to worry about everything that could happen

Under Eye: I can stay present in this moment

Under Nose: I can feel safe in this moment

Under Mouth: Releasing this story now

Collarbone: Allowing myself to feel safe now

Under Arm: Relaxing my mind and body now

Top of Head: Feeling calm and safe in the present moment

Take a deep breath, and check back in with your catastrophizing. How intense does it feel now on a scale of 0 to 10? Give it a number, and keep Tapping until you get the relief you desire.

DISRUPTING CONSTANT WORRYING

Worry, worry, worry—when will it ever stop? Even when your worrying doesn't qualify as catastrophizing, the act of worrying constantly can rob you of the opportunity to experience joy and be fully present in your life and with your children. Like most habits, though, even when you want to stop your constant worrying, it can be hard to control. That's because your brain has well-established neural pathways that support your worrying habit. Let's look at how to use Tapping, which sends powerful calming signals to the brain, to break the habit of constant worrying.

Tapping Exercise: Releasing Constant Worrying

Are you a "worrywart"? Do you go through your days constantly worrying about what *could* happen?

On a scale of 0 to 10, how intense and persistent does your worrying seem? Give it a number. For example, if you worry to the point that your worrying is interfering with your sleep and/or other parts of your health and well-being, you might rate the intensity of your worrying habit as a 9 or 10.

As you think of this, note a few of the things you worry about most often. Just jot down a few notes on them, or bring them to mind.

Now take 3 deep breaths. We'll begin by Tapping 3 times on the Karate Chop point:

Karate Chop *(Repeat 3 times)*: Even though I worry constantly, I deeply and completely love and accept myself.

Eyebrow: So many worries

Side of Eye: Always something to worry about

Under Eye: I can be a bit of worrywart

Under Nose: So much to be worried about

Under Mouth: All these worries

Collarbone: It's hard to stop worrying

Under Arm: There's always something else to worry about!

Top of Head: So many things to worry about

Eyebrow: All these worries

Side of Eye: I can't seem to quiet them

Under Eye: I can be such a worrywart

Under Nose: So many worries

Under Mouth: This worrying is exhausting

Collarbone: This worrying is distracting

Under Arm: I don't like worrying!

Top of Head: I can let go of these worries

Eyebrow: I can let myself feel safe

Side of Eye: Releasing these worries now from every cell in my body

Under Eye: Allowing myself to feel safe as a parent

Under Nose: Allowing myself to relax and release these worries

Under Mouth: It's safe to trust that my child is safe

Collarbone: I can focus on what's happening now

Under Arm: I can feel safe right now

Top of Head: Allowing myself to feel safe and calm now

Take a deep breath. How intense is your constant worrying now? Give it a number on a scale of 0 to 10, and keep Tapping until you get the relief you desire.

You can also try simply speaking your worries out loud or in your head as you tap. For example, *I'm so worried that she doesn't make friends easily... why won't she interact with other kids?... just so worried... she seems so afraid to play with them... I'm so worried... all this worry about her not making friends... I need to do something... I don't know what to do... all this worry... all this stress... it's weighing me down... she doesn't make friends easily... I feel like that's somehow my fault... is she not confident enough to make friends?... what have I done wrong?... all this worry... all this fear... so much shame and blame toward myself... maybe there's no rush... she's taking her time... that's okay... maybe I can stop blaming myself... and start relaxing... she'll make friends when she's ready... letting all this worry go... releasing this need to blame and shame myself about it... it's safe to trust that she'll make friends when she's ready... it's safe for me to stop worrying... and stop blaming and shaming myself about it... nothing's wrong, and I can let this stress and worry go now... I can let myself relax now... and trust that she'll make friends when she's ready... at the perfect time... it's safe to trust... and safe to let myself relax about this...*

BONUS EXERCISE: WHEN WORRYING PERSISTS

If the habit of constant worrying persists, try using Tapping as a tool for self-discovery. Tap through the points while asking yourself questions like:

- What's all this worrying really about?
- What would happen if I stopped worrying?
- Where in my life do I feel unsafe physically, emotionally, creatively or intellectually?

Whatever you discover, make a point of Tapping on it until you get the relief you're seeking.

RELEASING WORRIES THAT ARE TIED TO THE PAST

Ever since Jess broke her arm at the playground when she was 2 years old, her mother Robin experienced intense anxiety whenever they went to the playground. During each visit, Robin would hear herself constantly yelling to Jess to "be careful" and "watch out." Over time the playground had become a stressful place for both of them. Now almost 6 years old, Jess had grown increasingly moody at playgrounds, sitting on the bench even when her friends asked her to play with them.

Robin could see that her own fear of Jess getting hurt again was rubbing off on her daughter. But each time she saw Jess climbing, running or jumping on the playground, her mind flashed back to that day four years ago when her daughter had suddenly screamed in pain. During those first few seconds, Robin hadn't known how badly hurt Jess was. The terror she'd felt then still felt very real, but Robin didn't know how to let go of her fear and move on.

When past events have led to our children getting hurt in some way, it's easy to get into the habit of worrying that similar events will recur. The fastest way to let go of what happened is to tap through the original event. Once the emotional intensity of the memory is gone, you'll be able to release your worry and be more present in what *is* happening rather than what *could* happen.

Tapping Exercise: Releasing Worry—Will It Happen Again?

When you notice yourself worrying about whether a past event will recur, check in with yourself. How intense is the emotional charge you experience when you think of the original event? Give it a number on a scale of 0 to 10.

Next begin by Tapping through the points as you mentally walk through the original event silently in your mind or out loud. Since Tapping sends your brain calming signals, this exercise allows you to release the emotional charge of your memory.

Note: If at any point you encounter traumatic memories and feel overwhelmed, stop Tapping and seek the assistance of a qualified professional who can help you to use Tapping to release the trauma you experienced. For a list of EFT practitioners, visit The Tapping Solution EFT Practitioner Directory at http://thetappingsolution.com/eft-practitioners/ (and remember that many practitioners will work with you over the phone or via Skype, so they don't necessarily have to be local to you).

As you tap and tell yourself the story, remember any sights, sounds, smells, colors, textures and people you associate with the story's different parts.

When you reach the first point of emotional intensity in the story, as Robin did when she recalled hearing Jess wail loudly just after breaking her arm, tap just on that moment until you can recall it without experiencing an emotional charge. Once the emotional charge is gone, you can move forward in the story.

Repeat this process at each point of emotional intensity in the story. When you think you've released all the emotional charges, retell your entire story from beginning to end. If you notice any additional intensity, stop and tap through those points again.

Continue this process until you can retell the entire story, from beginning to end, without experiencing any emotional intensity.

> ### *BONUS EXERCISE:* DISRUPTING "BUT WHAT IF..."
>
> So many of our worry thoughts begin with the words "but what if..."
> When you hear yourself saying or thinking *but what if,* try Tapping through
> the points while speaking your *but what if* fears until they carry little to no
> emotional charge.

RELEASING WORRIES ABOUT YOUR RELATIONSHIP WITH YOUR CHILD

As your child grows older and more independent, you may also worry about changes in your relationship with him/her. For example, the sweet, open exchanges you had with your elementary-school-aged child may turn into defiance or silence once s/he enters middle school.

Although these parent/child relationship changes may be normal, they rarely feel that way. Understandably, you worry about the direction that your relationship with your child is taking. You may also worry whether your child will tell you if something's wrong, or if s/he is struggling at school, and so on.

Since children are likely to act out during these times of change and uncertainty, your worries may be compounded by their hurtful words and/or behavior. Whether your child begins to ignore you, or gets in the habit of yelling, "I hate you," you may feel overwhelmed by worry *and* a host of other challenging emotions.

By Tapping on your worries, as well as the other layers of your experience, you may not change your child's behavior or experience overnight, but you will be able to weather their emotional, mental and physical evolution with greater ease and peace of mind. As we've seen, that sense of calm alone can transform your own experience, and your child's as well.

Tapping Exercise: Releasing Worry about Changes in Your Child

Focus on an instance when you first noticed the changes in your child. Did you pick him/her up from school and suddenly get the silent treatment? Did s/he yell, "I hate you!" when you said no to a sleepover? Think back to a moment when you first noticed a significant change in their attitude and/or behavior.

When you think about that moment, what is the primary emotion you feel? Are you worried about your child? Do you feel angry about how s/he spoke to you or treated you? Do you feel overwhelmed by his/her new and unsettling behavior?

Be honest with yourself about how you're feeling. When you're ready, give that primary emotion a number of intensity on a scale of 0 to 10.

Take a deep breath, and begin by Tapping 3 times on the Karate Chop point:

Karate Chop *(Repeat 3 times)*: Even though I'm so overwhelmed and worried about these changes in my child, I love myself and accept how I feel.

Eyebrow: I'm so worried

Side of Eye: And so overwhelmed

Under Eye: I don't understand why this is happening

Under Nose: Why does my child suddenly seem so different?

Under Mouth: Is something wrong?

Collarbone: Is something happening at school?

Under Arm: I don't know what to do

Top of Head: I feel so powerless

Eyebrow: All this worry

Side of Eye: It's so stressful

Under Eye: And I'm so frustrated by how s/he's acting

Under Nose: Why is everything suddenly so different?

Under Mouth: Why is s/he suddenly so withdrawn/defiant/etc.?

Collarbone: What's going on?

Under Arm: I'm so worried about him/her

Top of Head: All this worry

Eyebrow: It's overwhelming

Side of Eye: I can let myself feel it all now

Under Eye: And I can let it go

Under Nose: I'm not sure how to handle this

Under Mouth: And that scares me

Collarbone: But that's okay

Under Arm: I can let it all go now

Top of Head: And I can relax when I think about these changes

Take a deep breath and check back in on your primary emotion, and any other emotions that might come up. Keep Tapping until you get the desired relief.

IDENTIFYING PATTERNS AROUND WORRYING

As you focus on what worries you most, you may begin to notice patterns. For example, you may realize that most of your worrying is about your children's grades, or about money or certain relationships. Maybe you worry most often in specific situations or around certain people. These are your patterns around worrying. Make a point of noticing them.

If you can release your worries, you will be better able to share your best self with your children—and when you do that, you'll also be teaching them that they, too, can be their best selves. It's a positive chain reaction that will cause ripple effects in your life and your children's lives now and for decades to come.

What are you willing to do differently? Will you tap daily? Get more sleep? Worry less and laugh more? Especially when we make them become new habits, the smallest changes often yield huge results. I can't wait to hear about yours!

Chapter 5

Reinventing Routinely Challenging Moments

What if, instead of looking at parenting as one enormous, ongoing experience, we look at it as a series of moments?

And what if, by learning to manage one moment differently, we could change the way we act and react in the next moment, and then the one after that, and on and on?

Just by handling that one moment in a new way, we could change our entire experience around parenting! Let's play with that idea, and look at some of the opportunities that present themselves.

TOUCHSTONE MOMENTS

Nearly every parent I've worked with has stories about the routinely challenging moments they experience with their children.

Maybe it's when they check their child's writing assignment and end up in (yet another) fight.

Or maybe it's at bedtime when their formerly sleepy children become suddenly energized and defiant.

As much as we, as parents, try to make these regular moments less stressful, the emotional and behavioral patterns they create quickly become a part of our lives.

What if, instead of seeing these moments as an inevitable part of parenting, we viewed them as opportunities for transformation? As different as these routine moments may seem externally, they have one thing in common—they all push our buttons. Whether we're being passively ignored or aggressively provoked, each of these moments creates in us some kind of emotional response that impacts the way we act and react.

These "push your button" moments often appear in one of two forms: when your buttons are pushed as a result of your child shutting down or withdrawing emotionally; or when your child is provoking you by testing your limits in some way.

In this chapter we'll look at how to use Tapping to create a new experience around the first type of "push your button" moments—when your child is struggling with their own emotions by shutting down or withdrawing emotionally.

QUIETING THE URGE TO "FIX" IT

Mary's 12-year old daughter, Kate, had just returned home from school. Usually talkative and energetic, today she was lying silently on her bed. She seemed bothered, "off" in some way, but not at all interested in talking about why.

Mary was concerned, and also unsure about what to do. Had something happened at school? Should she give Kate space, or try to get her to do some Tapping on how she was feeling? This wasn't their normal way of communicating. Mary had always made a point of creating space for the two of them to talk about their experiences and feelings.

A regular "tapper," Mary had tried to tap with Kate, but she'd always said it was "too weird." Nonetheless, Mary had seen Kate Tapping on her own in her room a few different times. That had been reassuring. Mary wanted more than anything for her daughter to have tools that would allow her to express and release her emotions, rather than holding them in, as Mary had done for so many years.

Tapping and meditation were such a part of their home, in fact, that when Mary was irritable or feeling off herself, Kate would remind her that it was "time to tap," or "time to go meditate, Mom." Mary felt grateful that she and Kate had been able to incorporate these tools into their relationship in such natural, lighthearted ways.

On this particular afternoon, however, Kate wasn't interested in communicating or Tapping. In fact, she seemed determined not to speak.

When I talked with Mary a few days later, she was still thinking about that afternoon. She still didn't know what had been on Kate's mind that day, and she still didn't know what, if anything, she needed to do about that.

Hoping to lessen the charge of that event, I asked Mary to visualize her daughter on her bed that day. I then asked her how she'd felt at that moment seeing Kate. Mary responded that she'd felt fearful. I then asked Mary where in her body she felt that fear. "In my chest," she replied. "It's an 8 out of 10."

As she tapped through the points, I asked Mary what that fear was about. "Funny how all of this stuff comes up when you're Tapping, huh?" she mused. We both laughed before she continued. "The fear is about when I was a child, and not being able to talk to my parents about anything. I just wish my parents hadn't been so busy. I wish they'd been more open to wanting to communicate, more willing to make some effort."

That remembered fear turned to sadness, as Mary regretted the distance in relationship with her parents. She began to cry as we tapped, using statements like, "Even though I feel all this sadness in my body, I choose to relax... Even though I feel all this sadness in my body, I couldn't communicate and that felt so sad, I love, accept and forgive myself."

We then tapped through the points using reminder phrases like, "Feeling all this old sadness in my body... Letting it go now."

After several rounds of Tapping, Mary's sadness had gone down to a 2 out of 10.

In just 10 minutes of Tapping, she'd found clarity on why she'd been so afraid about her daughter not communicating AND resolved the sadness from her childhood that she hadn't been consciously aware of until then.

GIVING THE GIFT OF COMMUNICATION

Like Mary, many of the parents I've worked with are committed to giving their children a different childhood experience than what they themselves had. Rather than avoiding and suppressing emotions, they want to allow their children to thrive in every way—academically, socially *and* emotionally, at school and at home. It's amazing and inspiring, and I'm deeply honored to be a part of their journey.

What I notice, though, is that as parents we're often misdirected by our desire to spare our children the pain that we experienced. Like Mary, we feel the urge to rush in and use Tapping (or meditation, etc.) to "fix" or remove any "bad" emotions our children seem to be experiencing.

However important Tapping and other mindfulness practices can be for children, it's also important for us, as parents, to notice how we're feeling when we're struck by an urge to spare our children from emotional pain.

We may find that oftentimes the goal of sparing our children pain is out of alignment with what we ourselves yearned for as children. Like Mary, many of the parents I've worked with suffered as children because they couldn't *communicate* about their emotions and experiences. They don't mourn the fact that they ever experienced fear, anger and other "bad" emotions. What they mourn as adults is the inability to communicate openly and lovingly with their parents.

Maybe our job as parents isn't to take away our children's
pain. Instead, maybe our job is to give them the gift of open and
honest communication.

Whether you use Tapping exclusively on your own or also with your children, remember that just by giving them the gift of open, loving communication, you are helping them to heal and allowing them to thrive.

#DOINGOOD

One day as I was thinking about how much parents are doing these days to help their children thrive, I stumbled upon an online video ad campaign that uses the hashtag #doingood. Released by Minute Maid, with whom I have zero association, it sums up perfectly the message I want to convey, which is this—you *are* enough, and you *are doing* enough.

Taking the time to use Tapping on yourself is a gift you're giving to your children. After Tapping, you will be more relaxed and centered, better able to listen to what they have to say, and more available to support them on their journeys. In other words, your own emotional availability and the open communication it creates with your children is, unto itself, a gift beyond measure.

Let me say it again—you *are* enough, and you *are doing* enough. When you come to parenting believing those two things, your entire experience will be transformed forever.

TRANSFORMATION BY EXAMPLE

One week after our 10 minutes of Tapping together, Mary called in with an update. She'd had several great, although somewhat surprising, experiences since our last call. While she hadn't had much time to do more Tapping herself, the shift she'd experienced that day had seemed to transform her entire household.

Since our last call, Kate had been coming home from school talking about all of the experiences she was having at school. Without any prompting, Mary's husband had also begun opening up to her more about what was happening with him at work. "It's been incredible!" she exclaimed, explaining that her own Tapping had allowed her to be more present at home.

By resisting her natural parental urge to rush in and "fix" the emotions Kate was feeling that afternoon, Mary gave herself the opportunity to express and release her own emotions. In doing so, she created an even larger opportunity for herself, her daughter and husband to move forward in a more positive way.

I've seen these kinds of transformations happen in people more times than I can count. It's a powerful testament to how much we can transform our lives, including our relationships with others, when we first take care of ourselves.

THE SECRET TO LASTING TRANSFORMATION

While it's impossible to say exactly how and why our own transformation so quickly "infects" people around us, some of that magic seems to lie in opening up to our own emotions. When we can do that, we can fully release them and be more present with others. That presence alone transforms our relationships.

In a culture that often judges emotions as "good" and "bad," allowing ourselves to feel and release emotions isn't always easy. From a young age many of us were taught to resist our emotions, especially the "bad" ones like fear, sadness and anger. Without realizing it, we learned to spend a lot of time and energy avoiding those emotions.

Think for a moment about how you respond to your own "bad" emotions. For instance, when you feel angry, do you hold it in and/or fear its destructive force? Do you let yourself feel deep sadness or do you push it away, maybe by trying to think positive instead? When you're afraid, do you tell yourself that you're "fine," or try to rationalize why you shouldn't feel afraid?

Most of us have subconscious patterns that prevent us from feeling the true force of our emotions. Unfortunately, by denying our emotions, we allow them to become more powerful, not less. Over time, these repressed emotions drain us of present-moment attention and energy.

In other words, denying ourselves the experience of our own emotions turns out to be a *lot* of work!

Wanting to spare our children of this burden, we may then feel an overwhelming need for them to share how they're feeling with us. When they don't, we may feel threatened, as Mary initially did.

By allowing ourselves to feel and release our own emotions, we create space for others. We become more present, and everyone around us, especially our children, quickly sense that.

Ironically, it is by tending to our own emotions and allowing ourselves to let go and feel more that we are finally able to create the space for our children to do the same.

So how can we allow ourselves to be more open to our own emotions? It begins with accepting ourselves *with* our emotions, including the "bad" ones. Let's do some Tapping on that now.

Tapping Exercise: Feeling Safe with Your Emotions

To begin, take a deep breath. On a scale of 0 to 10, how safe does it seem to feel "bad" emotions like anger, fear, sadness, guilt, regret, shame and more? If it helps, think back to a recent moment when you felt these emotions. Did you struggle to let yourself be angry, sad, guilt-ridden or other? If so, on a scale of 0 to 10, how resistant were you?

Now take a deep breath. We'll begin by Tapping 3 times on the Karate Chop point:

Karate Chop *(Repeat 3 times)*: Even though it doesn't feel safe to feel some of my most intense negative emotions, I love myself and accept how I feel.

Eyebrow: All of these strong emotions

Side of Eye: They don't feel safe

Under Eye: I can't let myself feel all of these emotions

Under Nose: They're so big

Under Mouth: They're so overwhelming

Collarbone: I don't have time to feel these emotions!

Under Arm: All of these emotions

Top of Head: It's all too much

Eyebrow: I can't let myself feel some of these emotions

Side of Eye: They're too big, too overwhelming

Under Eye: I can't let myself feel them

Under Nose: They hurt too much

Under Mouth: This doesn't feel safe

Collarbone: I can let myself feel them now

Under Arm: It's safe to feel these emotions

Top of Head: I can feel them when I'm Tapping

Eyebrow: It's safe to let myself feel these emotions now

Side of Eye: I can feel them when I'm Tapping

Under Eye: It's safe to feel all of my emotions

Under Nose: I can feel them now

Under Mouth: And let them go

Collarbone: I can let myself feel them

Under Arm: And I can let myself release them

Top of Head: It's safe to feel all of my emotions

Take a deep breath. If you think about feeling anger, sadness, guilt, fear and other negative emotions now, how resistant do you feel on a scale of 0 to 10? Keep Tapping until you feel safe experiencing these emotions.

As you begin to make peace with letting yourself feel the full spectrum of your emotions, you can then begin to focus on how to manage them when your child is struggling with his/her own. Let's take a look at how to do that next.

BEING PRESENT WITH VULNERABILITY

As a parent, there are few experiences that feel as raw as watching your child suffer. More than anything we want to take away their pain, save them from the hurt, sadness, anger and other emotions we've struggled with. As we've seen, though, sometimes the best thing we can do is be present with what they're feeling.

To do that, you first need to allow yourself to be vulnerable along with your child. Instead of trying to take away their vulnerability or avoid your own, you can be present with their emotions, as well as your own. This takes practice.

Let's do a 2-part Tapping exercise now to begin the process:

Tapping Exercise: Part 1–Gaining Peace Inside of Yourself

We'll begin this exercise by using Tapping to create a deep sense of calm and peace within yourself. Then, we'll focus on being present with your child as they process their own vulnerability. Think back to a moment when you were tempted to "fix" or remove challenging emotions your child was feeling. Whether it's fear on the first day of kindergarten or a troubled silence from a tween or teen, picture yourself in that moment. Now ask yourself:

- What emotion do I feel when I imagine this moment?

If you're unsure which emotion it is, you can also tap through the points while asking yourself that question.

Once you're clear on the primary emotion the image evokes in you, give that emotion a number of intensity on a scale of 0 to 10.

Then begin Tapping through the points and ask yourself more questions:

- Where in my body do I feel this <name your emotion>?

As you continue Tapping through the points, ask yourself a few more questions:

- What's this <name your emotion> all about?
- Where did this <name your emotion> come from?
- When did this <name your emotion> begin?

Use the answers to those questions as your Tapping targets.

For example, let's say your child is feeling sad, and you sense that her sadness is the result of overhearing the fight you and your ex-spouse just had. As you look more closely at how her sadness is making you feel, you realize that her sadness is causing you to feel an overwhelming sense of guilt.

As you tap, you then realize that your guilt creates a feeling of heaviness in your chest. You also remember overhearing your own parents fighting about how to parent you when you were a child. The guilt you feel about your daughter's sadness is actually stemming from old guilt you felt from "making" your parents unhappy.

Using all of this information, you could then do Tapping. Remember, there are no "right" or "wrong" ways to use Tapping, but to help you move forward, here's a sample Tapping script based on the scenario described above:

Karate Chop *(Repeat 3 times)*: Even though I feel so much guilt and sadness, it's been with me for so long, I love and forgive myself now.

Eyebrow: So much guilt

Side of Eye: So much sadness

Under Eye: These emotions have been with me for so long

Under Nose: So much old guilt

Under Mouth: So much old sadness

Collarbone: All this heaviness in my chest

Under Arm: It's safe to feel it all now

Top of Head: Letting myself feel it now

Eyebrow: All this old sadness

Side of Eye: All this old guilt

Under Eye: So much heaviness in my chest

Under Nose: I just couldn't make them happy

Under Mouth: So much old guilt

Collarbone: So much old sadness

Under Arm: All these old emotions

Top of Head: Letting myself feel them now

Eyebrow: So many old emotions

Side of Eye: It's safe to feel them now

Under Eye: And it's safe to let them go

Under Nose: It's safe to release them

Under Mouth: I can let them all go now

Collarbone: It's safe to let this all go now

Under Arm: Choosing to relax and feel safe now

Top of Head: Feeling at peace in mind and body

Take a deep breath. Give your primary emotion a number of intensity on a scale of 0 to 10 now. Keep Tapping until you get the relief you desire.

Tapping Exercise: Part 2—Being Present with Your Child's Vulnerability

If you've sufficiently cleared your issue, you'll begin to feel a sense of relief. From that place, you can support your child by being present with their vulnerability, rather than by trying to "fix" anything.

To begin that process, picture your child again in his or her vulnerable moment. What emotion does that evoke in you now? On a scale of 0 to 10, how intense is that emotion?

Continuing our example from Part 1, as a result of the Tapping you've done on releasing guilt, perhaps you now feel sadness that your child is sad. Instead of blaming yourself for it, you accept that your divorce is best for everyone, though you still feel sad that she's having to struggle with this sadness.

Use Tapping now to release this sadness. Once you've lessened the intensity of your own emotional response, you can be present with your child as they navigate their own emotional experience.

While there are countless ways to create space for your child to experience their own emotions, I wanted to share some of the different ways that the parents with whom I've worked have done that:

- Gave their child space, and did Tapping on their own.

- Sat with their child in silence as they cried or experienced their vulnerability in some other way.

- Used journaling to express themselves, individually or together, and then tapped through the points while repeatedly reading what they wrote until the journal entry held no emotional charge. (Again, our goal here is not to stop feeling emotions, but instead, to feel them fully, so that we can then let them go. When we do that, we can be fully present in the moment, rather than subtly distracted by repressed emotion from the past.)

- Listened to their child give voice to their emotions without expectation or judgment, and then thanked their child for sharing.

- Asked their child if they want to tap on whatever was bothering them, and then accepted their answer without question or comment.

- Did an art project together to express how they were feeling.

- Did some form of exercise or therapeutic art together—went on a hike, run, walk, did yoga, made music, painted, etc.

These are some of the many ways to be present with your child's vulnerability. Above all, trust your instincts, and when in doubt, tap on what you're feeling first.

Now that we've looked at how to manage your child's emotional pain, in the next chapter we'll take a look at the other kind of "push your buttons" moment—when your child seems to be testing your limits.

Chapter 6

Managing Conflict by Releasing Taboo Emotions

How many times have you said things like:

"It's time to do your homework."

"Clean up your room."

"Stay seated at the dinner table until you're done."

A simple but often repeated reminder—"time to get your pajamas on"—can turn into an ongoing pattern of stress that gets played and replayed. Every evening you anticipate the test of wills that's about to happen—and like clockwork, it does.

One of the most frustrating aspects of these moments is how powerless they make us feel. We try and try to get our children to change their behavior, but at the end of the day, we can't *make* our children listen. We can't *force* them to act differently.

So how can we transform a situation that we can't control? As we saw with Mary, by releasing our own emotions, we act and react differently. As a result, we can often transform a situation faster and with more ease than we ever imagined. Relaxing in the midst of a conflict can be hard to do, though, since in those moments we're often overwhelmed by frustration, irritation, anger and more. Let's look at how we can use Tapping to make that process easier and more effective.

ALLOWING A NEW RESPONSE TO EMERGE

Getting ready for school had been a challenge at Ana's house for some time. Every morning she'd gently awaken her 10-year-old daughter, Isobel. Hoping for the best, she'd ask Isobel to get dressed for school and go downstairs to prepare breakfast and lunch. Most mornings Isobel would ignore Ana's request and stay in bed. Occasionally, she'd come downstairs in her pajamas and cocoon herself in a blanket on the couch.

As the minutes ticked by, Ana's anxiety would quickly escalate. Glancing at the clock as she went through her morning routine, Ana would continually remind Isobel to get dressed. Once they'd reached the point when Isobel was about to be late for school, Ana's patience would run out, and she would start yelling at her daughter to get dressed. Isobel would eventually do as she was asked, but by the time Ana dropped Isobel off at school, they both felt exhausted and defeated. It was a stressful start to the day.

When Ana and I first began talking, she shared that she was in the midst of making several important life changes. Becoming a calmer and more confident parent was one of the changes she intended to make. The first step, she felt, was turning their morning routine into a more pleasant and peaceful experience. As committed as she was to making that change, however, she felt powerless to make it happen. She'd already tried numerous variations on their morning routine, but nothing had worked.

As we began Tapping, I asked Ana to envision their morning routine starting at the first point of tension. She shared that she usually woke up exhausted, dreading the nearly daily conflict with Isobel, as well as the busy workday ahead. As soon as she envisioned time passing with Isobel still in her pajamas, Ana began to feel a strong sense of panic in her body.

As we began Tapping on her panic, Ana began to cry. For years, she'd been running on fumes. Sleep-deprived, stressed about growing her new business and feeling unsupported as a single mom, she remembered one specific morning earlier in that same week. Once again, she'd been asking Isobel to get dressed for school when she suddenly felt all of her energy leave her body. She'd felt physically drained, unable to push anymore.

As she recalled that moment, Ana experienced that familiar sense of panic in her body. We did several more rounds of Tapping on feeling and releasing it.

Afterward, Ana shared that she felt like Isobel was hurting her by not listening. Every morning she asked Isobel to do the same thing—get dressed for school so they could leave the house in time. No matter how kindly or how often Ana asked Isobel to complete this simple, necessary task, Isobel continued to dawdle.

On a rational level, Ana knew that Isobel wasn't actually trying to hurt her. However, the experience always *felt* that way to her.

Let me say that again, because it's a common experience that's incredibly important. While Ana knew, on a rational level, that Isobel wasn't intentionally hurting her, Isobel's passive defiance *felt* intentional to Ana.

We've all had that moment when a negative experience or reaction from someone *feels* intentional. When you're in it, embroiled in a test of wills with your child, their behavior and their choices can *feel* personal, as if they're intentionally working against you.

When you step away from the moment, as Ana did while Tapping, it may be easier to acknowledge a more objective truth—that children are *supposed* to test our boundaries; that we all may need a healthier bedtime and sleep routine so we wake up more rested; and so on.

We often react to this kind of split reality experience, where your heart is saying one thing and your rational brain is telling you another, in one of two ways. Like Ana, you may give in to your emotional experience (by lashing out, for example). At other times, you may try to dominate and control your emotional experience. While the latter reaction may sound preferable, it's only a short-term fix. Eventually, your emotions will erupt, or work against you in some other way.

There is a third option that can provide long-lasting relief. Instead of unleashing your felt experience or trying to dominate it, you can express and release it in a safe way. That's where Tapping comes in.

LIFTING THE TABOO

Feeling negative emotions like anger and resentment toward our children isn't easy or straightforward. After all, it's our job to nurture, support and protect them. How can we feel anger or resentment toward them? These feelings are perfectly natural, but they don't sit easily within us.

How, then, can we shed our original negative emotions—anger, resentment or other—when we're being suffocated by guilt and shame for feeling those emotions in the first place? Sometimes the best way to release our emotions is to let them out by saying the words we wouldn't normally dare to speak. Let's use Tapping to do that now.

Tapping Exercise: **Releasing Taboo Emotions**

Before you begin this exercise, find a quiet, comfortable space where you won't be overheard or disrupted. We're going to be releasing intense emotions, so privacy, especially from your children, is important. Carve out enough time, at least 15 minutes, for you to complete this process.

When you're ready, think of a routine moment that leads to conflict of some kind. Maybe it's when you go to the mall and your child pitches a fit when you say no to buying him something. Maybe it's when your child starts playing with toys every time you ask her to clean up her room. Whatever it is, focus on that moment now.

Begin playing the scene through in your mind. What emotion do you feel most intensely when you think of it? Give that emotion a number of intensity on a scale of 0 to 10.

Begin Tapping through the points, beginning with the Karate Chop point, as you let yourself feel the anger or frustration or resentment you tend to feel in that moment. As you continue Tapping through the points, speak the words you'd say to your child if you let yourself unleash your emotions.

Remember, we're doing this in a safe, private space. To let your emotions go fully, you need to speak the words you've spent so much time and energy not saying. Since you'll be Tapping throughout the process, your brain will receive the signal that it's safe to relax, express yourself and then fully release whatever intense emotion(s) you're feeling.

As an example, let's say that Ana felt resentful toward Isobel while envisioning their stressed-out morning routine. In that case her Tapping might go something like this:

Karate Chop: (Repeat 3 times): Even though I feel all this resentment toward Isobel, and she won't get up and get going when we need to go, I love myself and accept how I feel.

Eyebrow: You're making everything so much harder

Side of Eye: Why are you always working against me?

Under Eye: Why won't you just listen?

Under Nose: You're making everything so much harder

Under Mouth: Things are hard enough

Collarbone: I don't need you making everything so much harder

Under Arm: Why do you have to work against me so much?

Top of Head: I'm so tired of yelling

Eyebrow: Why are you working against me?

Side of Eye: I just need you to get dressed!

Under Eye: You're making things so much harder

Under Nose: Everything's already hard enough

Under Mouth: I hate that I feel this way

Collarbone: So much guilt around feeling this resentment

Under Arm: So much shame around not being the parent I want to be

Top of Head: I'm tired of feeling this way

Eyebrow: It's safe to feel this resentment

Side of Eye: And it's safe to let it go now

Under Eye: All this resentment in my body

Under Nose: It's safe to feel it

Under Mouth: And it's safe to let it go now

Collarbone: Releasing all of this resentment now

Under Arm: Just letting it all go

Top of Head: Feeling calm and centered in my body now

Keep Tapping, saying everything you need and want to say. If the focus of your Tapping shifts from your child to someone else or some other event or part of your life, go with it! Continue Tapping until you've fully released the emotional charge of your negative emotions.

When you're ready, return to the original moment you tapped on. Run through that same scene in your mind until you can replay it from start to finish without experiencing any emotional intensity.

CONNECTING THE DOTS

As Ana and I continued to explore the layers of emotion around her and Isobel's morning routine, she came to an important realization. "This is the same pattern I've had in all of my relationships," she shared. "It's part of a long history of being in relationships with people who hurt me."

She then told me about multiple relationships in her past that had ended with her getting hurt. As she spoke, Ana realized that her past relationships with others had been distorting her relationship with Isobel. Since she'd always been hurt in other relationships, her subconscious mind was recreating that scenario with Isobel.

By the end of our Tapping, when Ana envisioned their morning routine again, her panic was gone. Instead, she felt frustrated, which was great progress. "It feels like a much healthier response to the situation," she explained. Knowing that she could use Tapping to quiet her frustration when it arose was also comforting.

As we wrapped up our Tapping session, Ana shared that although she was still sleep-deprived, she didn't feel as emotionally exhausted as she had before Tapping. That, too, was great progress.

Sometimes progress happens suddenly in one gigantic wave, and at others, it unfolds more gradually, one shift at a time. In the latter case, it's important to notice, as Ana did, that moving from panic to frustration is a significant and positive shift.

As she continues to tap through her frustration, she'll have an easier time relaxing, which will also give her more access to her creative brain. That's often where our big "Aha!" moments begin, and also where our best creative problem-solving happens. For Ana, that will support her in devising new approaches and solutions to weekday morning tension.

LIGHTENING YOUR LOAD

When we're Tapping through "push your button" moments, it's common to stumble upon bigger themes, as Ana did when she identified her past pattern of getting hurt in relationships.

These realizations by themselves can feel hugely powerful. Often we experience a profound sense of relief—*Aha! Finally I get it!* We tell ourselves that just *knowing* why we're feeling a certain way is such a huge step forward that we don't need to do any further Tapping.

While it *is* important to celebrate that progress, until you complete the process by Tapping through the root issue(s) you discover, you're still carrying the same heavy emotional load. Although you may have a clearer understanding of *why* you have that load, deep and lasting relief only becomes possible when you tap through the root issue(s) itself.

Oftentimes we avoid Tapping through the deeper root issue(s) that we discover because it doesn't sound like fun. Digging into dark, difficult emotions and memoires? *Uh, no thanks*, we say to ourselves. We've all been there, and we've all run in the other direction.

We may also avoid Tapping through root issue(s) because we've been told that it takes a long time. Once again, this is where Tapping is such a powerful tool. As we saw with Mary in Chapter 5, and I've seen with many thousands of others over the past 10-plus years, with Tapping it's possible to clear big issues from the past in 10 or 20 minutes.

That's a HUGE payoff in a very short period of time!

By spending just a few minutes Tapping, you can become that calmer, more confident parent Ana aspired to be.

Thanks to a few minutes of Tapping, home becomes a place of solace and connection, rather than conflict and stress.

With those minutes of Tapping, you can sleep better, communicate better and become more productive. You can feel healthier, happier and more sincerely positive about your life than ever before.

I hope you give yourself the gift of willingness. When you notice yourself resisting the opportunity to tap on deeper issues, start Tapping! Tap through the points while saying things like, "I don't feel like looking at this issue," and "Tapping on this doesn't sound fun," or "Tapping on this sounds boring."

Then imagine what it will feel like to wake up with an even deeper sense of relief, a lighter emotional load than you've known in years, even decades. Your entire experience around parenting *can* and *will* transform, and those changes can happen so much more quickly than you imagine.

In the next chapter, I'll show you exactly how simple and quick that process can be.

Chapter 7

A Fresh Look at Transforming Parenthood

A few months after she was diagnosed with a life-threatening health condition, Barbara's ex-husband initiated a vicious custody battle for their 12-year-old daughter. This meant that while her doctors were regularly warning her to avoid stress, which had likely caused her condition, her lawyers were delivering terrifying news about potential threats to the custody of her daughter.

To add to her stress, money was tight. At the recommendation of her lawyer, Barbara and her current husband had recently hired a second attorney. Her ex-husband was drawing her daughter into the custody battle, and Barbara had been advised that at 12 years old, her daughter would need her own legal representation.

I learned about all this on the first call for *The Tapping Solution for Parents Group*, my four-week "bare bones" program for parents. Like dozens of others, Barbara had submitted an application to participate in this program. She was one of the first people in the group to tap with me live online.

As soon as she began telling her story, I could hear the stress and strain in her voice. She was consumed by guilt, regret, anger and fear, and the stress of it all was taking a serious toll on her health. The results from her recent lab results had shown significant declines in her physical well-being, and her doctors' warnings about her future were growing increasingly severe. Due to the custody battle, however, she'd been suffering from chronic insomnia, which is known to increase physical, emotional and mental stress.

Since Barbara's health condition caused chronic physical pain and discomfort, I began by asking her if she was in pain at that moment. Rather than focusing first on external stressors, it's often best to start by listening to the body. It's our most reliable messenger, especially when trauma and/or emotional overwhelm are involved.

Barbara shared that she wasn't in pain at that moment, but that her neck felt extremely tight. The tension in that area was an 8 out of 10. We did several rounds of Tapping on that tightness, as well as the guilt, anxiety and regret she felt about her current situation.

After a few rounds, the tightness had moved from her neck into her shoulders. Shifts like these, especially with physical pain, are known as "chasing the pain," and they indicate that the body is responding to Tapping. In these cases, the pain (or other sensations, such as tightness, tingling, hot/cold, etc.) needs to shift and move before it dissipates completely with further Tapping.

When I asked Barbara which emotion was entangled with the tension in her shoulders, she responded that it was fear, both about losing her daughter, and about what her daughter was having to go through as a result of the custody battle. We continued Tapping through her fear, as well as the tightness in her shoulders. Barbara then shared that she'd felt unsafe for a long time. For years there had always seemed to be someone bullying, accusing or threatening her. The custody battle over her daughter was the latest example of that ongoing pattern.

As we continued Tapping, Barbara began to feel a release. For the first time in years, she could see that it might be possible for her to feel safe, even now. While her external circumstances weren't likely to change soon, she could tap through her fear and other emotions, and begin to trust that she was supported and safe.

By the end of our Tapping that day, Barbara felt like she'd released a portion of the worry and other emotions she'd been carrying. As we finished our Tapping, I asked if she'd be willing to continue Tapping on any physical pain or discomfort she experienced throughout that next week, between our sessions. She agreed to do that.

GETTING BIG RELIEF IN LESS TIME

When we're Tapping through emotions and experiences, we may notice underlying themes, which are core limiting beliefs that help shape who we are, how we parent, even how we live our daily lives.

Using Tapping to release these core limiting beliefs, and the emotions and events connected to them, we can experience major stress relief surprisingly fast. As we've seen, that relief then allows us to be more available as parents, and that presence then allows us to transform our experiences around parenting.

By now, you'll have noticed that one underlying issue we often see is a lack of safety—the core belief "I am not safe." Keep in mind that I'm using "safety" here in a broader sense, to describe threats to our emotional and mental well-being *as well as* threats to our physical selves.

Often since childhood, many of us have struggled with feeling safe in our bodies (due to disease, trauma, weight or other), in our relationships (due to disconnection, neglect, abuse or other), and in our work and finances (due to debt, lack of fulfillment or other).

As parents, of course, our focus on safety only increases. At any given moment, we face an endless list of challenges and concerns around keeping our children safe, not just from getting hurt but also from being left behind, bullied and more.

Above all, we want our children to feel the underlying sense of security that we perhaps never felt. As Barbara realized while Tapping, however, we can't pass down feelings of safety if we ourselves don't have them. And as we saw with Wendy in Chapter 4, when we don't feel safe ourselves, we're also more prone to "catastrophizing" worries.

Moving beyond Trauma

If you're struggling with trauma, whether it occurred recently or in childhood, I urge you to seek out support whenever possible. Even a few Tapping sessions with an EFT practitioner can transform your entire experience. You can find a list at http://thetappingsolution.com/eft-practitioners/.

Are there areas in your life where you don't feel safe? The first step to addressing core issues around lack of safety is noticing where they manifest for you. Let's use Tapping to do that next.

Exercise: Identifying Patterns around Feeling Safe

To begin, ask yourself these questions:

- Do I feel safe in my body?

- Do I feel safe feeling and expressing my deepest emotions?

- Do I feel safe when I have to make challenging parenting decisions?

- Do I feel safe when I think about my own childhood?

- Do I feel safe asking for help and support when I need it?

- Do I feel safe being seen and heard at home, work and in my relationships?

- Do I feel safe earning and managing money/finances?

If you feel stuck, anxious or other difficult emotions when reading this list, tap through the points as you answer the questions. Once you've identified the area(s) where you don't feel safe, make a note of them and continue Tapping on each one until they're fully released.

It's completely normal, even common, to discover multiple areas where you feel unsafe. If that's the case, tap through them one at a time. You'll be amazed at how much you can release by Tapping for just a few minutes each day.

NEW ENERGY CREATES NEW LIFE

3 weeks later, Barbara called a second time. It was our fourth and last group call, and she was excited to be able to touch base one more time. Right away I noticed how different she sounded. Her voice was much clearer and more energetic.

When I asked her how she was doing, she replied, "I am doing much better, thank you… [Tapping] has made such a difference in the past 3 weeks, even to the point where my husband has made positive comments about Tapping!"

Barbara then explained that the external stressors in her life—the custody battle, her health condition, and financial limitations—were all still there. None of it had magically gone away. In spite of it all, though, she *felt* completely different. The constant worrying and mental chatter that had always plagued her had quieted considerably. Whenever it did flare up, she started Tapping.

While Barbara was still concerned about her daughter and the custody battle with her ex-husband, she was having an easier time trusting her lawyers to do their job. It had been a theme during the past 3 weeks, she added. For the first time in many years, she was noticing herself letting go of things, people and situations that she couldn't control. Many of the physical symptoms of her health condition had also subsided substantially.

I love stories like this. Here was Barbara just 3 weeks later, living the same life, managing the same external stressors, wrestling with the same amount of uncertainty, and yet her entire outlook and daily life had been transformed.

These improvements in her well-being hadn't enabled her to halt the custody battle, but they had allowed her to be more present and available to take better care of herself and her daughter. That alone is huge!

Over time, if she continues Tapping, I have no doubt that these internal transformations will lead to further external results—in her health, relationships, finances and beyond.

Barbara was just one of many parents who experienced significant relief after a relatively small amount of Tapping. Next let's look at how Mary's transformation changed her home life.

SMOOTHER DAYS, DEEPER CONNECTIONS

A couple of weeks had passed since Mary and I tapped on releasing the sadness about her relationship with her own parents. Since our call, she'd gotten into the habit of Tapping daily. She'd often tap at different times throughout the day, just whenever she felt stressed or noticed her "mental chatter" starting. She'd been amazed by the difference it had made. Even her busiest days seemed to flow more smoothly.

One big difference had been with her family's weekday mornings, which, like Ana's, had long been a source of stress. Since Mary had begun Tapping, however, her family's mornings had become calmer. It was Kate, her middle-school-aged daughter, who first noted the change. Recently, out of the blue, she'd thanked her mom for being more available to talk with her on weekday mornings. It had made a big difference, she said, to be able to share her thoughts and feelings with Mary before heading off to school.

Their weekday early morning conversations had been rewarding for Mary as well. Her relationship with Kate felt closer than ever, and Mary knew it was because she herself was far less stressed. Since beginning to use Tapping more often, she'd also been sleeping more soundly, and was waking up feeling more alive and energized than she had in a while.

Mary's husband had also benefitted. On a recent early morning, he'd accidentally backed his brand new truck into the garage. Not wanting to wake her up, he'd tapped on it instead.

Later that day he called her and shared how much Tapping had helped him to calm down. "I'm amazed at how much better I was able to handle it and not get stressed about it!" he'd said. A few days later, he texted Mary a note of appreciation:

> Over the past couple of weeks, you've been even calmer than usual. Thank you for that. You're my rock and my inspiration and you make me want to be a better person.

Laughing as she shared with amazement how much Tapping had impacted her entire family in just a few weeks, she added that she'd originally joined the group to find out how to tap with Kate. "I was hoping to find a way to tap with her so she didn't dismiss it as too weird." What ended up happening, though, was that she, and then her whole family, had been transformed. All 3 of them were now Tapping, and their communication and interactions as a family had improved as a result. "It's been incredible!" she added.

IT'S ALL INTERCONNECTED

Although we're often encouraged to compartmentalize our lives—conditioned to expect that work happens (mostly) at the office, personal life at home and so on—the reality is our lives are our lives. We can't shut off that side of ourselves when our kids aren't in front of us. Similarly, when we're stressed about relationships, money or work, that stress impacts our mood, patience, energy level and, by extension, our parenting.

> *Regardless of how our time is structured,*
> *the different parts of our lives are intricately intertwined*
> *on emotional and mental as well as logistical and financial*
> *levels. As a result, any time we spend Tapping on releasing*
> *emotions, memories and stress has a positive ripple effect*
> *on our parenting, our relationships with our children*
> *and how our home life functions.*

Deanna was also experiencing a positive ripple effect in her life. Having recently begun divorce proceedings, she was having to transition abruptly from being a work-when-she-could mom into a full-time working mom. Without her husband's full financial support, she needed to grow her coaching/teaching business significantly within a short period of time to support and care for herself and her four children.

Since the first *Parents Group* call, she'd been Tapping on her limiting beliefs about herself. As a result, she'd been feeling calmer, more energized and positive about the future than she expected to feel so soon after beginning her divorce. She'd also been more relaxed and available to her four children, which was helping them to navigate the divorce process as well.

Let's use Tapping to look at your own core beliefs about yourself, since transforming them is an essential part of lasting transformation.

Exercise: Examining Core Identity Beliefs

Since we'll be looking at your core identity beliefs, it's important not to filter yourself. Before you begin, carve out some quiet time and space to reflect on your current beliefs about who you are.

Take 3 deep breaths to ground yourself in your body and the present moment.

Either on paper or out loud, without overthinking it, finish this sentence:

I am _____.

Notice what comes to mind when you complete the *I am* statement. What does it say about how you feel about yourself in these aspects?

- as a parent
- at home
- at work
- in your body
- in your family
- financially
- in an intimate relationship

In this process most of us uncover some negative, limiting beliefs we have about ourselves. These are your Tapping targets. Be sure to tap through each one individually, but know that you don't need to do this in one sitting or one day or even week. Just move through them one at a time, being sure to clear each one fully before Tapping on the next one.

While completing these *I am* statements, you may also discover positive beliefs about yourself, and if so, great! Tap those in as often as possible. After Tapping on releasing limiting beliefs and negative emotions, Tapping in the positive is a great way to get a boost.

Since beliefs tend to be deeply rooted in experience as well as emotion, they may require repeat Tapping. Often a few minutes a day over a few days or weeks is sufficient.

Congratulations! You've successfully completed Part 1. Whether you've noticed a series of small changes or a massive shift, I hope that you keep Tapping. As you do, the momentum you've gained will increase and produce even more positive shifts in your experience.

Now that you've had some experiences with Tapping yourself, it's time to look at how to tap with your child. That's what we'll do next, in Part 2.

PART TWO

Tapping with Children

Chapter 8

How to Tap with Children

The first question I typically hear from parents is, "How do I use Tapping with my child?" It's a great question that has a million answers, depending on your child's age, mood and present-moment interests.

Let's look at some ways to bring Tapping into your home with the most ease and effectiveness.

COMMON CHALLENGES REGARDING TAPPING WITH CHILDREN

Here are several of the most common challenges I hear from parents:

"My child won't sit still!"

One of the benefits of Tapping is that it doesn't require stillness. In fact, it's the opposite—Tapping *requires* movement. You can tap while sitting, standing, walking or jumping around. If your child can't stay still, move along with him/her as s/he mimics you as you tap through the points alongside him/her.

"My child thinks it's a game."

With older and younger kids alike, I encourage parents, whenever possible, to allow for Tapping to feel light and fun. Since its purpose is to relieve the body, heart and mind of stress and heavy emotions, Tapping doesn't need to feel serious to be effective. If your child thinks Tapping is a game, go along with it. Intentionally making Tapping into a game can also be a great way to get younger kids to try Tapping.

"My child thinks I'm tickling him/her."

If your child collapses into a fit of giggles because your Tapping on him/her feels ticklish, that's fine. Laughter is powerful stress relief! Let him/her enjoy that moment, and if necessary, avoid the ticklish Tapping points next time.

"I can't get to all of the Tapping points."

Parents who tap on their kids often say that they can't get to all of the points. Especially with younger kids, it can be challenging. Again, let your child be comfortable and tap on any points you can reach, even if it's just one.

"He/she says Tapping is too weird."

Since children spend more time and energy on fitting in as they get into their middle- and high-school years, anything "weird" can be a tough sell. Try suggesting Tapping on something your child wants—better sports performance, less worry about friends or whatever it may be for them. For younger kids, you can also demonstrate by Tapping on a favorite stuffed animal or doll.

If your child remains resistant to Tapping, don't force it. Instead, lead by example and use Tapping yourself. As we saw in the first part of this book, children often notice and appreciate positive changes in your mood, energy, and attention. Over time those positive changes may make your child more open to trying Tapping on him- or herself.

"We tapped once, but I can't get them to try it again."

If your child has had an experience with Tapping, but isn't interested in doing it again, trust that you've planted a seed that will yield further results when your child is ready.

In the meantime, if you feel anxious about your child's unwillingness to do further Tapping, tap on it! As we saw in the first section of this book, the more stress relief you give yourself, the more you and your entire family will reap the rewards.

"We tried Tapping, but it didn't work."

Tapping sometimes produces immediate, dramatic results, and at other times it leads to only gradual, incremental changes. Feeling a little better, a little more relaxed, a little less afraid, etc. means that Tapping is having a positive impact at a more moderate pace.

"I keep trying, but my child won't let me tap on him/her."

Some kids may prefer to tap on themselves, which is great! Tap along with your child, and have him/her mimic your movements. If your child wants you to tap on the points for him/her, but doesn't like certain points, avoid those and stick to whichever points s/he doesn't mind you Tapping on.

"There are so many issues to tap on, I don't know where to start."

Throughout this book, there are numerous case studies of kids who are facing multiple major challenges at school and at home. Wanting to give them relief, we, as adults, may want to tap with them on bigger issues. It's critical, however, not to push children too far. Especially when kids are facing major challenges, the best entry point is through the present moment.

For example, if an elementary school child who's struggling with his or her parent's divorce is frustrated because a friend won't play the game s/he wants to play, focus your Tapping only on her/his present-moment experience—frustration about the game. Tap with her or him on immediate-need issues like this as often as s/he is willing, but don't try to push him or her to do Tapping on his or her parent's divorce unless, and until, s/he wants to.

This same principle applies to older children, as well. If a middle school or high school child is stressed out about a test, tap on that test anxiety. If s/he also wants to discuss and tap on social challenges s/he is facing at school, wait to tap on those when s/he is willing.

As always, if your child is resistant to Tapping at times when you feel s/he needs it, be sure to do Tapping yourself to release any stress, fear or worry you may feel as a result of her or his resistance to Tapping. The more negative energy you shed, the more available you can be for your child. That's hugely helpful to him/her as well as to you.

Introducing Tapping to Children

When you're ready to introduce Tapping to your child, the best approach is to keep it simple. This basic 3-step process can be tailored to different age groups:

1. Share a brief story of how the brain and body work together, in a relatable way. (Full details are numbered below. Rest assured, there's no need to become a neuroscientist!)

2. Explain how Tapping impacts the brain and body.

3. Use Tapping to help your child solve a problem *s/he* wants to solve.

Note: If you're new to Tapping, begin by reading Chapter 2. Tapping is simple to use and learn, but you do need to have a working knowledge of how to do it yourself before you introduce it to your child.

You can also visit the following link to watch a brief video on how to tap: http://www.thetappingsolution.com/#how-to-do-eft-tapping.

Let's look at what the process of introducing Tapping looks like for different age groups.

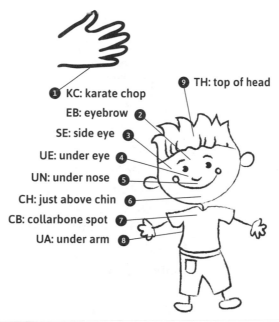

1. KC: karate chop
2. EB: eyebrow
3. SE: side eye
4. UE: under eye
5. UN: under nose
6. CH: just above chin
7. CB: collarbone spot
8. UA: under arm
9. TH: top of head

Tapping with Elementary-School-Aged Children:

Kids grow up and mature quickly, so two kids who are only two grades apart may approach and understand learning differently. As much as possible, tailor each step to your child's specific interests, desires and learning style.

When first showing your child how to tap, select a calm moment when s/he is able to focus. You can offer to show her/him a fun game, or frame it as a game that's really healthy for your brain and body. Again, the goal here is to keep things light and fun, and to get children interested on *their* terms.

Once your child is willing to learn more, keep the process straightforward. Here are a couple of examples of what that could look like.

1. **First, explain how the brain & body work together...**
   You, as the parent or adult, could say something like:
   Example 1: *You know when you feel sad (or mad) because a friend won't play a game with you, and you can't stop feeling that way because it almost feels like that sad (or mad) feeling is in your body? That's because your brain and your body are working together to create sad (or mad) feelings.*

Or, you can refer back to a time when they felt an emotion they wanted to overcome, but couldn't:

> Example 2: *Remember at John's birthday party when all of your friends were having so much fun swimming in the big kids' pool, but you were like a statue at the edge of the pool? Remember how you were too scared to go in, even though you really, really wanted to? Well, when things like that happen, your brain and body are working together to create scared feelings in your body.*

2. **Second, explain how Tapping impacts the body...**
    Example 1 (cont'd): *The fun part is what we call magic Tapping points on the body. When we tap on them gently, we can get rid of the sad (or mad) feelings when we don't want them.*
    Example 2 (cont'd): *The great thing is we all have magic Tapping points on the body that can get rid of that scared feeling.*

3. **Third, use Tapping to solve a problem they're interested in solving...**
    Examples 1 & 2 (cont'd again): *How about we try using our magic points? It's fun! It's a little like playing Simon Says where you follow what the other person is doing. Watch me, and tap on your body in the same places, okay?*

If your child is interested in continuing to tap, you can either tap on a topic s/he wants to tap on, or just keep Tapping through the points as you talk or answer questions. If you end up in a fit of giggles, even better. You've just given your child a positive first experience with Tapping!

Gorilla Thumps & Other "New" Points

In his children's book, *Gorilla Thumps & Bear Hugs*, my brother, Alex Ortner, gives parents an easy way to introduce Tapping to younger children. One of the many things I love about his book is how he renames some of the Tapping points in ways that appeal to younger children. Here are his names for them:

Standard Tapping Point Names	*Child-Friendly Tapping Point Names*
Karate Chop point	Karate Chop point
Eyebrow point	Hairy Eyebrow point

Side of Eye point	Super Eagle Eye point
Under Eye point	Lion Cry point
Under Nose point	Dragon Fire point
Chin point (or Under Mouth)	Wolf's Chin point
Collarbone point	Gorilla Thump point
Underarm point	Bear Hug point
Top of Head point	Monkey point

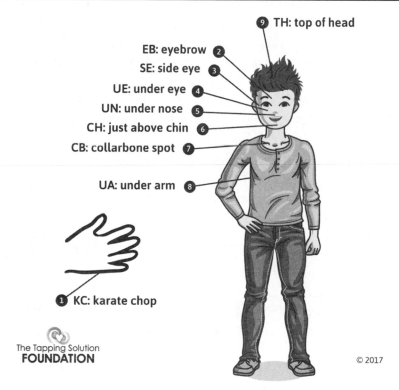

⑨ TH: top of head

EB: eyebrow ②

SE: side eye ③

UE: under eye ④

UN: under nose ⑤

CH: just above chin ⑥

CB: collarbone spot ⑦

UA: under arm ⑧

① KC: karate chop

The Tapping Solution
FOUNDATION

© 2017

Tapping with Middle-School-Aged Children:

This is a challenging age for kids and parents alike. Often kids are more physically developed than they are emotionally mature. They're also expected to meet more expectations at school and home, while simultaneously investing more of their time and energy into fitting in socially and gaining greater independence from family.

When trying to introduce your middle school child to Tapping, you once again want to appeal to them through their interests and desires—to score more in sports, have an easier time with homework, feel more like they belong or whatever it may be for them.

1. **First, explain how the brain & body work together...**
   Appeal to your child's experiences, frustrations and goals. For instance, you could say something like...
   Example: *Remember that time when you were angry with <best friend> and you couldn't stop thinking about it? (Or that time when you got so nervous before the big game that you felt like you didn't play your best? Etc.) Well, that happens because when you feel stressed out or upset, your brain tells your body to release something called cortisol.*
   When there's a lot of cortisol in your body, your feelings of stress or upset can get stuck in your body. So even when you want to stop thinking or feeling something, it's really hard to. Does that make sense?

2. **When your child is ready, explain how Tapping impacts the body...**
   If your child is interested in mindfulness, you can frame Tapping in those terms, since Tapping is a way of practicing mindful awareness of emotions and the body.
   Example (cont'd): *There's this technique called Tapping that sends calming signals to the brain. It's pretty cool, actually. By calming the brain, it also lessens the amount of cortisol in the body. When that happens, you feel better (or more focused, calmer, etc.).*
   You tap on these certain points on your body, and the bad feelings you don't want go away faster. So, for instance, by Tapping before a big game, you might end up playing your best because you feel less nervous.
   What's even better is that you can use Tapping in your room, or even in a bathroom stall right before a test. It really helps. Can I show you how it works?

3. **Third, use Tapping to solve a problem your child is interested in solving...**
   Ideally, at this point, you will tap along with your child on an issue s/he selects. If s/he is unwilling to tap, you can also demonstrate Tapping, using an example that's relevant to her/his interests. This will at least plant a seed for someday when s/he comes to you and asks about that "weird Tapping thing."

Example (cont'd): Let's say you're nervous about a big game or test and maybe you can't sleep the night before because your mind is racing and your belly aches. At bedtime you can start Tapping through the points as you say everything you're feeling stressed out about...

As you demonstrate Tapping, try to keep the mood light. If it feels right, go ahead and laugh with your child about the fact that Tapping looks weird. The truth is, Tapping *does* look weird. Now that we deeply and completely love and accept ourselves, though, we don't care about that anymore!

Note: If your child prefers, he/she can also watch this video to learn how to tap: http://www.thetappingsolution.com/what-is-eft-tapping/.

Tapping with Teenagers (High School):

While teenagers often need as much or more support than ever, they're also prone to rebel. In other words, teenagers often look and sound like a walking, talking paradox.

Again, the only thing you can do is plant a positive seed by introducing your child to Tapping. Don't force the issue, and always lead by example. If s/he notices how much calmer, happier, more confident you are as a result of Tapping, those positive changes will go a long way!

The first step of the process, of course, is to show and tell your child about it. Here's a simple but powerful way to do that:

1. **First, explain how the brain & body work together...**
    As always, refer to your child's interests and goals whenever possible. You may also want to include more science with this age group. Example: *Remember when your mind went blank while taking that math test? Well, there's a process that happens in the body called the "stress response" or the "fight or flight response." When you get stressed, a part of your brain called the amygdala tells your body to release a large amount of cortisol, which is called the stress hormone.*
    When there's a lot of cortisol in your body, it's hard to function normally. Your brain can "freeze" like it did that day when you couldn't think during your math test. That happens because stress is not just in your head, it's in your body, too.

If your child has questions about the amygdala and cortisol, try searching for "fight or flight response" and checking out some educational web sites together.

2. **Second, explain how Tapping impacts the body…**
Again, if your child is interested in mindfulness, feel free to frame Tapping in those terms.
Example: *There's this technique called Tapping that I've been learning about… It lowers cortisol levels in the body so you can think more clearly and your body can function better. It helps with test taking, releasing emotions like anger, sadness and others. It improves performance, whether in sports, theater and more. It also helps you fall asleep, and promotes better, faster healing in the body.*
You can use Tapping the night before your next math test, or whenever you want to feel more relaxed. You tap through a series of special points on the body—acupressure points from ancient Chinese medicine—while expressing and releasing stress and emotions. Want to try it?

3. **Third, use Tapping to solve a problem your child is interested in solving…**
Example: *Whenever there's something bothering you, or even when you want to sleep better or feel more focused or positive, a few minutes of Tapping can really help. Try it with me? Here's how it works…*

As always, your best leadership is by example, so tap on any anxiety or stress you're feeling as often as you can. If your child notices positive changes in you, s/he may eventually express interest on her/his own terms.

Measuring Progress

With all of the following Tapping techniques, whenever possible, it's best to begin your Tapping by measuring the intensity of whatever event, emotion or belief you'll be Tapping on.

For younger children, you can use the "this much" method of measurement, which is the most intuitive way for younger children to express how intensely they feel something. Spreading each arm open to each side, they can demonstrate the "this much" intensity of a given experience. As one example, if a child says s/he is mad, and opens his/her arms as wide open as s/he can, that would indicate s/he is feeling very, very mad. If s/he opens her arms halfway, that might mean she's mad, but not really, really mad, and so on.

For older children, you can rely on the 0 to 10 scale of intensity, with 10 being the most intense experience a child can imagine and 0 being no emotional charge at all.

TAPPING TECHNIQUES YOU CAN TRY WITH YOUR CHILD

Once you get comfortable with the basics of Tapping with your child, you may want to try some new Tapping techniques. Below are several techniques that you can keep in your Tapping "toolbox" to try with your child whenever it feels right.

> ### TAPPING TIP:
>
> When possible, start (and end) your Tapping with a deep, calming breath. Have your child notice and feel their breath moving in and out of the body.

"Tell the Story" Technique

This is great for releasing the emotional charge of past events and memories, and can also be used to dispel fears related to "what if" scenarios. Here's how it works:

- For this technique, you can skip the setup statement ("Even though I...") and instead begin Tapping through the points as you listen to your child tell the story of their memory, fear-based "what if" story, dream/nightmare or other.

- When they get to the first point in the story with an emotional charge, ask them to stop and rate the intensity of that moment, either on a 0 to 10 scale or using the "this much" method of measurement.

- Focus your Tapping on just that moment of the story until its intensity has decreased significantly or they get the desired relief.

- Continue Tapping, and have your child begin the story at the beginning again. If they can get to that first point of intensity in the story without feeling a big emotional charge, have them continue telling their story past that first point of intensity.

- If, while retelling the story from the beginning, your child reaches a second point of intensity, stop them again and repeat the same process you did for the first. Once that second moment has been neutralized, again have them start from the beginning.

- Repeat this process as many times as you need to. When your child can tell their entire story from start to end without experiencing significant emotional charge at any point, congratulations! You've successfully tapped through the story. Ideally, you'll want to do this process in one sitting; but if that's not possible, do as much as you can, and then keep going at another time, knowing that you may need to backtrack each time.

"The Box" Technique

If a child is struggling with trauma or other issue(s), this technique is a powerful way to give him or her relief without forcing them to face issues before s/he is ready and willing. By providing safe, protective distancing, and respecting your child's boundaries, it can also help to build and strengthen trust.

If you sense your child is shutting down or doesn't want to tap on an emotion or issue, ask him/her to imagine a box as s/he taps through the points.

As s/he continues Tapping, have her/him visualize the size, shape, color, and texture of the box. Is it a thick, sturdy box, or a cardboard box? Fill in as many details as possible.

Once the box appears very real in your child's mind, have him/her place the issue or emotion inside the box.

While continuing to tap, have your child imagine closing the box, the issue or emotion safely tucked away inside. When this image, and the issue or emotion it contains, feels safe inside, you can put the box away and save it for another time.

The next day, week, month, or whenever you feel is right, ask your child to recall that box again. While Tapping through the points, have him/her visualize opening the box. Ask your child if s/he is willing to tap through the contents. If not, respect her/his wishes and try again some other time. If s/he is willing, tap through the contents until s/he gets the desired relief.

Note: Especially for smaller children, it can be helpful to draw or design the box that s/he is going to put the issue or emotion inside. Art can be therapeutic, so if Tapping intersects with creating, that's great!

"The Box" technique is an important way of building trust with your child. That's also why it's essential not to push a child to tap through an issue or emotion until s/he is willing. If you feel worried or anxious because your child is resistant to Tapping on an issue for a long period of time, tap on it! Once you've done that, it will likely feel easier to trust that the safe container you've helped your child to create will eventually lead to a deeper healing process.

Visualization Technique

This technique is great for goal setting, releasing fears and overcoming limiting beliefs. Here's how to use it:

For younger children:

- This technique can be as simple as Tapping through the points while visualizing your fears floating away in a bubble. Or your child's fear might attach to a kite and fly away as you tap through the points together. Pick any visualization that appeals to your child.

- Add details to the visualization. For example, it might be a "pink, happy bubble," or a "magic, sticky kite that attaches to the scary feeling." Keep it simple, but relevant to their likes and dislikes, as well as their comfort and safety zones.

For older children:

- Have your child visualize something they'd like to achieve—acing a test, playing their best in a big game, performing, etc. As you tap along with them (or on them), have them notice any sensations they feel in their body, as well as any emotions they may feel when they think about that goal or desire.

  ○ For example, if your child wants to ace a test, but feels clenching in their stomach when they think about it, start by Tapping on that tight, clenching feeling in their belly, and then on their fear.

- Whenever possible, move from bodily sensations (clenching in the belly) to emotions (fear) to beliefs ("I won't ace the test because I'm not good at math"). Tap on each level of their response to visualizing their goal or desire until each one has been neutralized.

- When your child can run through the visualization and envision the desired outcome without experiencing a negative emotional charge, they'll likely have an easier time moving forward, whether by putting in more focused studying, practicing more or getting a restful night's sleep!

Visualization Technique with Colors

This technique can help younger children who don't always feel comfortable verbalizing their emotions to tap on and release them.

For example, if your child is struggling to verbalize how they're feeling, you could ask questions like:

If the way you're feeling right now were a color, what color would it be?

Is there a place in your body where you feel that <color> most?

Note: As always, when Tapping with your child, tailor your words to your child's age and experience.

If, for example, your young child says s/he feels red and it's mostly in her/his belly, you could then tap with her/him like this:

Karate Chop *(Repeat 3 times):* Even though I feel all of this red in my belly, I'm a great kid and I'm okay!

Eyebrow: All this red in my belly

Side of Eye: So much red!

Under Eye: All this red in my belly

Under Nose: I can feel it!

Under Mouth: That's okay

Collarbone: I'm a great kid

Under Arm: And I can let it cool down now

Top of Head: Maybe this red can turn to pink...

You can keep Tapping until the red has turned into a calmer, more neutral color.

SUCCESSFULLY TAPPING WITH YOUR CHILD

Now that you've learned more about the Tapping techniques you can use with your child, let's look at one of the most important things you can do to help your child experience successful emotional release with Tapping: capturing his/her experience and Tapping on that.

For example, if you want your child to focus on completing an assignment, and s/he is angry that you're interrupting her/his play or call with a friend, etc., focus the Tapping you do with your child on her/his anger at being interrupted, *not* on your desire for her/him to focus.

Let's be honest here—that is *really* hard to do when you're overwhelmed by your own emotions! That's also why it's so important for you, as a parent, to tap on releasing your own emotional experiences first before Tapping with your child.

Even after Tapping on your own, however, it may be tempting to tap with your child on what you want him or her to do, such as focusing on the assignment that's due. It's an understandable impulse, since an important part of your job as a parent is to teach your child any number of important lessons.

The reality is, though, if your child is distracted by emotions, s/he will struggle to hear what you're saying. By using Tapping to create space for emotional expression and release, you and your child can more successfully assume those roles—you as a guide and nurturer, and your child as a (sometimes) willing recipient.

> *Put simply, Tapping is not meant to be used as a parenting tool. Instead, it's a tool for emotional processing and release. Once that happens, you and your child can communicate better and complete any necessary tasks.*

In this example, that would mean *not* using Tapping to convince your child to focus. Instead, you would tap with your child on feeling and releasing his/her anger at being interrupted. Once that emotion has been quieted, your child may be more receptive to your parenting.

In other words, when you're Tapping with your child, it's *really* important to focus on *his/her* present-moment experience, even when that means not Tapping with your child because s/he doesn't feel like it!

A NOTE ON THE NEGATIVE... AND A LOT MORE ON THE POSITIVE!

As we saw in Chapter 2, the typical sequence with Tapping is to begin by focusing on releasing the negative, and then instilling the positive. With kids, this rule can apply, but not always. It's often a great idea to move quickly to the positive rather than dwelling on the negative. Depending on your child and the situation, you could also skip Tapping on the negative altogether, and focus your Tapping only on the positive.

Below are a couple of examples of what that might look like when, as one example, you're Tapping on your child's fear of the dark.

To address the "negative," but only briefly, you could say something like...

Karate Chop *(Repeat 3 times)*: Even though I get that scary feeling when it's dark, I'm an awesome kid and I'm safe!

Eyebrow: That scary feeling

Side of Eye: I get it in the dark

Under Eye: I can't see what's around me

Under Nose: That scary feeling

Under Mouth: I don't like it

Collarbone: That's okay

Under Arm: I'm a great kid

Top of Head: And I'm safe & sound!

Keep Tapping on the positive until your child gets the desired relief.

Or, you can skip the "negative," and move directly to the positive...

Karate Chop *(Repeat 3 times)*: I'm a great kid and I'm okay, even when I'm in the dark.

Eyebrow: I'm a great kid!

Side of Eye: I'm safe

Under Eye: I'm safe in the daytime

Under Nose: And safe in the dark

Under Mouth: I'm a great kid!

Collarbone: And I'm okay

Under Arm: Safe in the day

Top of Head: And safe in the dark!

Keep Tapping on the positive, associating safe feelings with the darkness, until your child gets the desired relief. If Tapping only on the positive doesn't provide sufficient relief, try some Tapping on the negative along with the positive, and/or experiment with other Tapping techniques.

Great! You're now ready to introduce Tapping to your child. If you feel anxious or unsure, try doing more Tapping on yourself. When you feel confident, your child will pick up on that confidence and be more willing to follow along.

After showing your child how to use Tapping, you'll be ready to look at how to tap on specific issues your child is facing. That's what the rest of Part 2 is all about. Feel free to pick and choose topics according to which challenges your child is facing on any given day.

Chapter 9

"Disorders": Specific Help for the Child with Specific Needs

TAPPING WITH YOUR CHILD: ADD AND ADHD

When you're using Tapping with a child who has ADD or ADHD, the best place to begin is by focusing on relieving the symptoms that these disorders cause. From inattention, hyperactivity and impulsivity to social anxiety and more, using Tapping on these issues separately has helped many parents offer their children significant relief.

As always, the first step is Tapping on yourself. Since these disorders create stress for parents, we'll start by Tapping on the stress and anxiety you may feel as a result of your child's ADD or ADHD. Once you've found some relief, you'll be ready to try Tapping with your child.

Adult Tapping: **Relieving Stress from Your Child's ADD or ADHD**

When you think about your child's ADD or ADHD and how it impacts your lives, how much stress do you feel on a scale of 0 to 10? Give it a number now.

Next, take a deep breath.

Let's begin by Tapping 3 times on the Karate Chop point:

Karate Chop (*Repeat 3 times*): Even though I feel all this stress because of my child's disorder, I deeply and completely love and accept myself.

Eyebrow: All this stress

Side of Eye: All this anxiety

Under Eye: I wish I could make it all go away

Under Nose: I wish I could make this disorder go away

Under Mouth: I hate that s/he has it

Collarbone: And I hate how stressed it makes me feel

Under Arm: I feel guilty for even saying that

Top of Head: It's so stressful

Eyebrow: All this stress

Side of Eye: So much I have to anticipate

Under Eye: So many challenges we face because of this disorder

Under Nose: I wish I could make it go away

Under Mouth: So much stress

Collarbone: I can let myself feel it now

Under Arm: And I can let it go

Top of Head: Letting myself feel this stress now

Eyebrow: And letting it go

Side of Eye: Releasing this stress from every cell in my body

Under Eye: Letting myself relax now

Under Nose: It's the best thing for everyone

Under Mouth: Releasing this stress now

Collarbone: Letting it all go

Under Arm: Feeling quiet and calm in my body now

Top of Head: Fully relaxing my mind and body now

Rate your stress now, and keep Tapping until you get the desired relief.

Now that you've had an experience, let's look at how to use Tapping with your child to relieve the symptoms of ADD and ADHD.

Note: As always, when Tapping with your child, tailor your words to your child's age and experience.

Overcoming Social Anxiety

Jon had been struggling ever since starting his first year of middle school. Diagnosed with ADHD during elementary school, he had grown increasingly overwhelmed by the social pressures he felt at his new school. The stress and anxiety were distracting him from schoolwork, and his grades had suffered as a result.

Noticing his growing angst, his mother asked if he'd be willing to tap with her. Although reluctant at first, he later agreed to try it. They began by Tapping on the social anxiety he was experiencing, as well as his fears around not fitting in.

He shared that some of the kids had been teasing him during recess. They continued Tapping on how he'd been feeling, as well as some of the times when he'd felt ostracized. After several rounds, his body and demeanor relaxed noticeably.

During the following year, Jon and his mom continued to tap together a few times per week. Very soon after they began Tapping together, Jon's mom noticed that he was in a better mood after school.

Over a period of months, his friendships improved, as did his grades. He's now doing well in school and has formed very close friendships with some of his new classmates.

Child Tapping: Overcoming Social Anxiety

If there's a specific situation your child is struggling with, have them tap through the points (or tap on the points of their body for them) while asking them about what was happening and how it made them feel.

Have them tell and retell the story while Tapping until they can tell the story from beginning to end without feeling anxious.

If your child has a general social anxiety that they'd like to tap on, start by asking them to rate how anxious they feel about social situations, either on a scale of 0 to 10 or using the "this much" method of measurement.

Then begin by Tapping 3 times on the Karate Chop point:

Karate Chop *(Repeat 3 times)*: Even though I feel nervous and uncomfortable when I'm around other people, I'm an awesome kid and I'm okay.

Eyebrow: I don't like being around other people

Side of Eye: It makes me feel nervous

Under Eye: It makes me feel uncomfortable

Under Nose: I don't like how it makes me feel

Under Mouth: It makes me nervous

Collarbone: Other people make me anxious

Under Arm: It feels icky

Top of Head: That's okay

Eyebrow: I'm a great kid!

Side of Eye: And people like me

Under Eye: I'm great at being me

Under Nose: And I'm great at being a great kid

Under Mouth: People like me as I am

Collarbone: I can let go of the icky feeling I get around other people

Under Arm: I feel calm and happy around other people

Top of Head: I'm a great kid!

Eyebrow: I'm okay

Side of Eye: I'm a great kid

Under Eye: And I can feel calm and okay around other people

Under Nose: I'm a great kid

Under Mouth: And I'm okay!

Collarbone: I can feel calm and okay around other people

Under Arm: I'm a great kid!

Top of Head: People like me, and I'm okay

Ask them to rate their anxiety (or "icky" feeling, etc.) about being around other people. Keep Tapping until they get the desired relief.

If their anxiety persists, there may be more specific issues that you need to tap on, such as:

- They're anxious about being around certain people. If so, tap through the points as you talk about why, and what happened to make them anxious around those individuals or groups. Keep Tapping until they get the desired relief.

- They have specific fears about not being liked, getting lost in a crowd or other issues that play into their social anxiety. Do some Tapping on those issues specifically. Keep Tapping until they get the desired relief.

Attending a New School (and Navigating Other Big Changes)

A school counselor recently shared a story that shows the power of Tapping with kids, including those who have survived tremendous hardship at very young ages.

It was the start of a new year, and Matt, a 2nd grader, had just begun attending a new school. Diagnosed with ADHD, he was having a hard time with the mid-year adjustment. In addition to acting out at school, he'd been unable to sit still in class and was falling behind with his schoolwork.

Unsure how to handle his disruptive behavior, Matt's new teacher reached out to the school counselor, who learned that Matt was living with his older sister and brother-in-law. They had recently become his new guardians. Prior to that, Matt had lived with his paternal grandmother. Both of Matt's biological parents suffered from substance abuse and had never been in his life.

After meeting with his guardians, who were previously unaware of Tapping, the school counselor received permission to try Tapping with Matt. His new guardians also shared that although he'd previously been on prescription medications to manage his ADHD, they were eager to try alternative methods. Matt's recent annual physical exam had indicated that he was in good health.

Given her heavy caseload, the school counselor explained that she would only be able to work with Matt on his school-related issues. His family history and traumas would need to be managed through a private practitioner.

When he first met with the school counselor, Matt was very willing to try Tapping, and talked openly about his dislike of school. When asked about his feelings, he explained, "It's hard to sit still and I don't like getting into trouble at school." At the start of their Tapping, his dislike of school and of getting in trouble was an 8 out of 10.

The counselor began by leading him through two rounds of Tapping on his dislike of school, which quickly dropped to a 5 out of 10. Since his dislike for getting into trouble hadn't yet dissipated, she then led him through several more rounds, using phrases such as:

- "I don't like school"
- "I hate getting into trouble at school"
- "It's hard to sit still and finish my work"
- "I'm a good kid"

When they were finished Tapping, the intensity of his feelings about school had gone down to a 1 out of 10.

At the end of the session Matt was smiling. "I like these exercises!" he said. He then asked if he could tap in his classroom. The school counselor encouraged him to tap on his finger and face points while he was at his desk to help him focus and sit quietly.

The counselor gave him a homework assignment—to share what he learned with his teacher and guardians, and to tap at home before bedtime and on his ride to school each morning. His teacher was also encouraged to allow him access to a "quiet Tapping spot" that was set up in the back of the classroom.

After a week of individual sessions, Matt was Tapping regularly in his classroom. He is now having more successful days than difficult days in school. He is no longer getting sent to the office and is on grade level academically in all subjects.

Child Tapping: Navigating Change

When your child is struggling with major changes, whether because of a new school, changes in home life or other, focus your Tapping on whatever they're struggling with in the moment. Rather than trying to solve the "bigger picture" of what's going on in their lives, focus on the present moment. By addressing these "present moment" issues, you can lower their stress and, over time, allow them to adjust more smoothly.

The first step is to zero in on what they're experiencing now. For example, if they're having a meltdown, you might do some Tapping with them on the anger or frustration they're feeling. If they can't settle down enough to focus on learning, tap on their inability to sit quietly to learn.

When you're clear on their present-moment issue, ask them to rate its intensity on a scale of 0 to 10, or using the "this much" method of measurement.

In this Tapping script, I'll focus on having trouble sitting still, but as always, tailor your words to your child's present-moment experience.

To begin, take a deep breath, and begin by Tapping 3 times on the Karate Chop point.

Karate Chop *(Repeat 3 times)*: Even though I can't sit still and I have to keep moving, I'm a great kid and I'm okay.

Eyebrow: I can't sit still

Side of Eye: I have to keep moving

Under Eye: I hate getting in trouble for it!

Under Nose: I can't sit still

Under Mouth: It's not my fault

Collarbone: I can't sit still

Under Arm: That's okay

Top of Head: I'm a great kid!

Eyebrow: So hard to sit still

Side of Eye: I don't like getting in trouble for it

Under Eye: I can't sit still

Under Nose: It's okay

Under Mouth: I'm an awesome kid!

Collarbone: I can feel calm now

Under Arm: Everything's okay

Top of Head: I'm a great kid

Eyebrow: I'm okay!

Side of Eye: I can feel quiet and calm inside now

Under Eye: I can slow my brain down

Under Nose: I can feel quiet in my body now

Under Mouth: I can feel silence in my body

Collarbone: I can slow my brain down now

Under Arm: Feeling calm inside

Top of Head: Feeling calm and quiet in my body and brain now

When they're ready, ask your child to rate how they're feeling now. Keep Tapping until they get the desired relief.

Child Tapping: Overcoming Inattention

If your child is struggling with focus, skip the rating stage and have them start Tapping through the points, or tap on them, getting to as many points as you can. Tapping is incredibly forgiving, so even Tapping without speaking can quickly reverse inattention.

When you're able, begin by Tapping 3 times on the Karate Chop point:

Karate Chop *(Repeat 3 times)*: Even though I can't focus right now, I'm a great kid and I'm okay.

Eyebrow: My brain is jumping around

Side of Eye: I can't pay attention

Under Eye: My brain is jumping around everywhere

Under Nose: My brain won't stop jumping around

Under Mouth: That's okay

Collarbone: I'm a great kid!

Under Arm: And I'm okay

Top of Head: It's okay that my brain is jumping around

Eyebrow: I can let it jump around now

Side of Eye: And I can let it calm down now

Under Eye: I'm a great kid!

Under Nose: I can do anything I put my mind to

Under Mouth: I can quiet my brain down now

Collarbone: I'm okay!

Under Arm: I can feel quiet in my brain now

Top of Head: And calm in my body

Eyebrow: I'm a great kid!

Side of Eye: I can do anything I put my mind to

Under Eye: Feeling quiet in my brain now

Under Nose: Feeling calm in my body now

Under Mouth: I'm a great kid!

Collarbone: And I'm okay

Under Arm: I can do anything I put my mind to

Top of Head: Feeling calm and quiet now

If your child is willing to rate their inattention now and compare it to what it was before Tapping, have them do so, either using the 0 to 10 scale or the "this much" method of measurement. Keep Tapping until they get the desired relief.

Child Tapping: Overcoming Impulsivity

If your child is willing to rate their urge to do whatever comes into their mind, have them give it a number on a scale of 0 to 10 or using the "this much" method of measurement.

Then begin by Tapping 3 times on the Karate Chop point:

Karate Chop *(Repeat 3 times)*: Even though I feel like I have to do things right away, I'm a great kid and I'm okay.

Eyebrow: All these ideas

Side of Eye: They come to me all the time

Under Eye: I have to act on them

Under Nose: All these ideas

Under Mouth: I have to act on them

Collarbone: I can't control it

Under Arm: All these ideas

Top of Head: I have to act on them

Eyebrow: That's okay

Side of Eye: I'm a great kid!

Under Eye: And I'm okay

Under Nose: So many ideas

Under Mouth: They come to my brain

Collarbone: I can let them stay there

Under Arm: I can feel quiet when they come to me

Top of Head: I'm a great kid!

Eyebrow: And I'm okay

Side of Eye: I can feel calm inside

Under Eye: Even when the ideas come to me

Under Nose: I can feel quiet inside

Under Mouth: Even when an idea comes to me

Collarbone: I'm a great kid

Under Arm: And I'm okay

Top of Head: Feeling quiet and calm inside now

Have your child rate their impulsivity now, either on a scale of 0 to 10 or using the "this much" method of measurement. Keep Tapping until they get the desired relief.

TAPPING WITH YOUR CHILD: SENSORY PROCESSING DISORDER

By sending calming signals to the brain, Tapping can help to moderate some of the symptoms of Sensory Processing Disorder (formerly known as Sensory Integration Dysfunction). Especially when Tapping is used on a regular basis, it can provide significant relief.

Since SPD can also cause significant anxiety and stress for you as a parent, as always, the best starting point is Tapping on yourself. We'll do that first and then look at some of the ways you can use Tapping with your child.

Adult Tapping: Relieving Stress from Your Child's SPD

When you think about all of the planning and energy you put into helping your child manage his or her SPD, how much stress do you feel on a scale of 0 to 10? Give it a number.

Take a deep breath.

We'll begin by Tapping 3 times on the Karate Chop point:

Karate Chop *(Repeat 3 times)*: Even though I feel anxious, stressed out and exhausted by my child's SPD, I love myself and accept myself.

Eyebrow: All this stress

Side of Eye: Always trying to anticipate how SPD will play out

Under Eye: All the worry

Under Nose: All the "what ifs"

Under Mouth: So stressful

Collarbone: It's exhausting

Under Arm: All this stress and anxiety around SPD

Top of Head: Sometimes it feels like SPD is running our lives

Eyebrow: All this stress around SPD

Side of Eye: All this worry about how SPD is impacting her/his childhood

Under Eye: All this anxiety about whether I'm managing it right

Under Nose: So much stress

Under Mouth: All this anxiety

Collarbone: Not sure I can't take it anymore

Under Arm: Maybe I can release it now

Top of Head: Letting myself feel this overwhelm now

Eyebrow: And letting myself release it now

Side of Eye: Everything's okay

Under Eye: And I'm doing everything I can

Under Nose: Letting myself relax now

Under Mouth: Releasing this stress from every cell in my body

Collarbone: Feeling calm and safe

Under Arm: Letting myself feel fully relaxed now

Top of Head: Feeling relaxed and at peace now

Take a deep breath, and check back in on the stress, anxiety and overwhelm you're feeling. Give it a number on a scale of 0 to 10 now. Keep Tapping until you get the desired relief.

Now that you've had an experience, let's look at how to use Tapping with your child.

Note: As always, when Tapping with your child, tailor your words to your child's age and experience.

SPD & Adjusting to a New School

Starting a new school can be overwhelming for any child, and even more so when that child also struggles with SPD.

When James became overwhelmed in kindergarten, his mother, a holistic health counselor, taught him Tapping. Although James had previously been diagnosed with Sensory Processing Disorder, she had chosen not to emphasize the label, which she felt was limiting.

From that point forward, they used Tapping at bedtime each night. Some nights James wanted to tap on the noise during recess or difficulties he'd had in class. There were other times when they tapped on releasing sadness from feeling rejected by classmates or falling behind in his schoolwork.

Often, they would finish by Tapping on James' intention to have a good day the following day and have fun playing with friends.

As a result of this nightly Tapping with his parents, James has adjusted to his new elementary school and kindergarten classroom with far more ease than he had previously. He rarely has a bad day at school anymore and is having a great time with his new school friends.

James is also becoming increasingly independent with his Tapping, and seems to find comfort from knowing that he can use Tapping whenever he's having a difficult time.

In cases like these, the simple act of Tapping regularly from a young age may have positive ripple effects that last a lifetime. Rather than pushing away bad experiences at school or with friends, he's able to release them through Tapping and then move to focusing on having another good day tomorrow. That small nightly shift sets him up for success each and every day. Awesome!

Child Tapping: **Adjusting to a New School or Environment with SPD**

If your child is focused on one new element of his or her new school, like the noise at recess, have him or her rate the "icky" feeling about that issue. If it's a general "yucky" feeling about everything being new, have him or her rate that. In either case s/he can use the 0 to 10 scale or the "this much" method of measurement.

I'll focus on the many new sources of overwhelm your child might experience, but as always, tailor your words to your child's experience if mine aren't relevant.

Begin by Tapping 3 times on the Karate Chop point:

Karate Chop *(Repeat 3 times)*: Even though I have such a big "icky" feeling about my new school, I'm a great kid and I'm okay.

Eyebrow: All these icky feelings

Side of Eye: I really don't know about my new school

Under Eye: So much new stuff

Under Nose: All those kids

Under Mouth: So much noise

Collarbone: All the colors

Under Arm: It's too much

Top of Head: I need it to stop

Eyebrow: Too much

Side of Eye: I feel so icky and yucky about all of it

Under Eye: I don't want to go

Under Nose: I just don't like it

Under Mouth: This icky, yucky feeling

Collarbone: Feeling it now

Under Arm: That's okay

Top of Head: I'm a great kid

Eyebrow: And I'm okay!

Side of Eye: I can let go of this icky, yucky feeling

Under Eye: I'm a great kid!

Under Nose: And I'm okay

Under Mouth: I'm a great kid at home

Collarbone: And a great kid at my new school

Under Arm: And I'm okay

Top of Head: I'm a great kid and I'm okay!

When your child is ready, have him or her rate the "icky, yucky" feeling again. Keep Tapping until s/he gets the desired relief.

Child Tapping: Overcoming the Need for Excessive Stimuli

If your child is unable to settle down because s/he is constantly seeking out new and more stimuli, it may be easiest to skip the rating stage.

If s/he won't sit still for Tapping, try moving around while you tap together. There's no pressure to stay still or seated while Tapping!

Start by Tapping 3 times on the Karate Chop point:

Karate Chop *(Repeat 3 times)*: Even though I always want more to do, more to see, more of everything, I'm a great kid and I'm okay.

Eyebrow: I want to keep going

Side of Eye: And doing more

Under Eye: Seeing more

Under Nose: I don't like being told to settle down

Under Mouth: I like to keep going

Collarbone: I don't like being told to calm down

Under Arm: It's frustrating

Top of Head: So much energy in my body

Eyebrow: That's okay

Side of Eye: I'm a great kid!

Under Eye: And I'm okay

Under Nose: I can have quiet energy now

Under Mouth: I can be a little calmer now

Collarbone: I'm a great kid

Under Arm: And I'm okay!

Top of Head: I can feel a little quieter now

Eyebrow: I'm a great kid

Side of Eye: And I'm okay

Under Eye: I can let myself feel quieter now

Under Nose: I'm an awesome kid

Under Mouth: And I'm okay

Collarbone: I can be calmer now

Under Arm: I can feel quieter now

Top of Head: I'm a great kid and I'm okay

If your child is quiet enough to talk about how s/he feels now, have her or him rate her/his feelings. If possible, notice if s/he feels a little or a lot quieter than before. Keep Tapping until s/he gets the desired relief.

Child Tapping: Overcoming Sensory Intolerance

If your child struggles with sensory intolerance, whether it's human touch, the feel of clothing, noises, certain tastes or textures, try using Tapping on the experience s/he can't tolerate. If there are several, pick one that feels most intense right now.

As always, tailor your Tapping to your child's specific issue, whether certain noises, tastes, textures or other.

To start, ask them to rate their icky feeling around the sensory experience you'll be Tapping on, either on a scale of 0 to 10 or using the "this much" method of measurement.

Let's begin by Tapping 3 times on the Karate Chop point:

Karate Chop *(Repeat 3 times)*: Even though I don't like this <sensory experience here>, I'm a great kid and I'm okay.

Eyebrow: I don't like <sensory experience here>

Side of Eye: It's yucky

Under Eye: This <sensory experience here>

Under Nose: I really don't like it

Under Mouth: That <sensory experience here>

Collarbone: It's icky

Under Arm: I don't like it

Top of Head: That's okay

Eyebrow: I'm a great kid

Side of Eye: And I'm okay

Under Eye: I don't like <sensory experience here>

Under Nose: That yucky <sensory experience here>

Under Mouth: That's okay

Collarbone: Even when I think of <sensory experience here>

Under Arm: I can feel quiet inside

Top of Head: I'm a great kid

Eyebrow: I can let go of how yucky <sensory experience here> feels

Side of Eye: I can relax when I have <sensory experience here>

Under Eye: I'm an awesome kid!

Under Nose: And I'm okay

Under Mouth: I can feel calm when <sensory experience here>

Collarbone: I can feel quiet inside when <sensory experience here>

Under Arm: I'm safe when <sensory experience here>

Top of Head: And I'm okay

When your child is ready, have him or her rate the icky feeling again. Keep Tapping until s/he gets the desired relief.

Child Tapping: **Overcoming Social/Emotional Issues Related to SPD**

If your child experiences anxiety in social situations, whether due to fear of being rejected, having trouble interacting or playing with other kids or any other issues, Tapping can help to calm your child's nervous system and help him/her be more at ease in social situations.

First, ask your child to think about a social situation—school recess, going to playdates, etc.—that makes him or her feel anxious (or icky/yucky), either on a scale of 0 to 10 or using the "this much" method of measurement.

Then begin by Tapping 3 times on the Karate Chop point:

Karate Chop *(Repeat 3 times)*: Even though I feel icky and yucky when I think about being with other kids, I'm a great kid and I'm okay.

Eyebrow: All those kids

Side of Eye: It gives me that icky, yucky feeling

Under Eye: What if they won't play with me?

Under Nose: What if they don't like me?

Under Mouth: This icky, yucky feeling

Collarbone: It makes me want to push

Under Arm: It makes me want to yell

Top of Head: All those kids, it's too much

Eyebrow: That's okay

Side of Eye: I'm a great kid!

Under Eye: Not sure about all those kids

Under Nose: Not sure they'll like me

Under Mouth: Not sure they'll play with me

Collarbone: That's okay

Under Arm: I'm a great kid

Top of Head: And I'm okay!

Eyebrow: I might have fun!

Side of Eye: I can play no matter what

Under Eye: I can have fun when I want to

Under Nose: I'm a great kid

Under Mouth: And I'm okay

Collarbone: I can have fun when I want to

Under Arm: I'm an awesome kid

Top of Head: And I'm okay!

When your child is ready, have him/her rate that icky, yucky feeling (or anxiety, nervousness, etc.) on a scale of 0 to 10 or using the "this much" method of measurement. Keep Tapping until s/he gets the desired relief.

Child Tapping: Introducing a Sensory Object/Experience

If your child continues to struggle with a sensory object or experience, you can also try introducing it with this exercise.

By using Tapping as well as protective distancing, you can allow your child to get comfortable with that sensory object/experience more gradually.

The goal with this exercise is to slowly get closer to the sensory object or experience while Tapping on your child's resistance at each step.

If you're Tapping on a sensory object, try to have that object physically present.

Step 1: Tapping at a Distance

As an example, if your child resists the feeling of clothes on his or her skin, you could begin by standing in front of his or her closet together.

Begin Tapping together while looking at the clothes hanging inside (or opening a drawer and looking at the clothes in there).

As you continue Tapping together, ask your child how he or she feels when s/he looks at the clothes in that closet or drawer.

If your child seems comfortable and calm when s/he is looking at the clothes, start with one round of positive Tapping and then move on to Step 2 of this exercise.

As an example, that positive round might look something like this:

Karate Chop *(Repeat 3 times)*: I'm a great kid, and I can feel safe and calm when I look at these clothes.

Eyebrow: These clothes

Side of Eye: I can feel calm when I see them

Under Eye: It's safe to feel quiet inside when I see them

Under Nose: These clothes

Under Mouth: I can feel calm inside when I look at them

Collarbone: It's safe to feel safe when I look at these clothes

Under Arm: I'm a great kid

Top of Head: And I can feel quiet inside when I look at these clothes

If your child feels anxious or resistant when s/he is looking at the clothes, ask him/her to rate how anxious, icky, etc. s/he feels, either on a 0 to 10 scale or using the "this much" method of measurement.

Then you can begin by Tapping 3 times on the Karate Chop point.

Karate Chop *(Repeat 3 times)*: Even though I don't like looking at these clothes, and I don't like how they will feel on my skin, I'm a great kid and I'm okay.

Eyebrow: These clothes

Side of Eye: I don't like how they feel on my skin

Under Eye: These clothes

Under Nose: I don't want to have to wear them

Under Mouth: These clothes

Collarbone: I feel anxious looking at them

Under Arm: These clothes

Top of Head: I don't like how they feel on my skin

Eyebrow: These clothes

Side of Eye: I'm really not sure about them

Under Eye: These clothes

Under Nose: Maybe I can relax when I look at them

Under Mouth: These clothes

Collarbone: I'm just looking at them

Under Arm: These clothes

Top of Head: Maybe they're not so bad

Eyebrow: I can look at these clothes

Side of Eye: I can feel calm when I see them

Under Eye: It's safe to feel quiet inside when I see them

Under Nose: These clothes

Under Mouth: I can feel calm inside when I look at them

Collarbone: It's safe to feel safe when I look at these clothes

Under Arm: I'm a great kid

Top of Head: And I can quiet inside when I look at these clothes

Take a deep breath. Ask your child to rate his/her resistance to looking at the clothes again. Keep Tapping until s/he is willing to have you move the clothes closer to him/her, whether on the floor, bed, or other.

Step 2: Tapping at a Closer Proximity

Once your child is willing to be closer to his or her clothes, move them as s/he continues to tap.

Ask your child to rate their anxiety or icky, yucky feeling about the clothes again, either on a scale of 0 to 10 or using the "this much" method of measurement.

Then continue by Tapping 3 times on the Karate Chop point.

Karate Chop *(Repeat 3 times)*: Even though I'm not sure about these clothes being so close to me, I'm a great kid and I'm okay.

Eyebrow: These clothes

Side of Eye: They're closer to me

Under Eye: I don't like that

Under Nose: I don't like how they feel on my skin

Under Mouth: These clothes

Collarbone: I don't like how they feel on me

Under Arm: I don't want them closer

Top of Head: I like them farther away from me

Eyebrow: I like it better when they don't touch me

Side of Eye: These clothes

Under Eye: Not sure about them getting closer

Under Nose: I don't like how they feel

Under Mouth: I don't want to wear them

Collarbone: I won't wear them

Under Arm: I don't like how they feel

Top of Head: That's okay

Eyebrow: I'm a great kid!

Side of Eye: I can feel safe being closer to these clothes

Under Eye: I can feel calm inside when I'm closer to them

Under Nose: I can quiet inside when I'm near them

Under Mouth: It's safe to feel safe when I'm near these clothes

Collarbone: I can relax in my body when I'm nearer to these clothes

Under Arm: I'm safe around these clothes

Top of Head: I'm a great kid and I can feel calm now

Take a deep breath together. Ask your child to rate his or her anxiety (or icky, yucky feeling, etc.) about the clothes now. Keep Tapping until s/he is willing to touch the clothes.

Step 3: Making Contact

Since it's important to continue Tapping as your child is touching the clothes (or other object), in this step you might drape the clothes on your child's back or leg.

Ask them to rate how anxious or resistant s/he feels about the clothes touching her/him, either on a 0 to 10 scale or using the "this much" method of measurement.

Take a deep breath and continue Tapping, as we've done in the previous steps.

If it's true to your child's experience, tap on his or her resistance—*these clothes feel icky on my skin… I don't like them touching my skin… they scratch me…* and so on.

Then gradually transition to positive statements… *I can feel calm when these clothes touch my skin… these clothes protect my skin… I can feel quiet inside when I touch these clothes… these clothes protect my skin… these clothes can help my skin…*

Keep Tapping until your child feels comfortable and calm with the clothes touching his/her skin.

When your child is ready, ask him or her to put the clothes on. (If s/he is still resistant, return to Step 3 and keep Tapping on the clothes touching her/his skin.)

Step 4: Full Contact

Once your child is wearing the clothes, continue Tapping on their resistance and then on feeling safe and calm with the clothes on. Keep Tapping until s/he feels calm wearing the clothes.

Congratulations! If you've made it to this point, you've successfully completed this exercise and helped your child to overcome his or her resistance to that sensory object!

If you're using this exercise for overcoming a sensory experience…

To use this exercise for overcoming a sensory experience, use the same process of gradually introducing the experience.

If you're unable to recreate the entire experience, try using video, photos, and/or your imagination to recreate the experience as fully and accurately as possible, integrating as many real-life sensory components—touch, sound, feel, etc—as you can.

Tap through each step, and before progressing to the next step, always get your child's okay first, and be sure to stop if s/he asks you to. You can always return to this exercise at another time when s/he is willing.

As one example, if your child becomes agitated in crowds...

- As Step 1, you could do some Tapping while watching a video of lots of people (or you can "paint" a picture of a crowd out loud or remember a time when s/he was in a crowd).

- In Step 2, you could add audio that sounds like a crowd of people and tap until your child is comfortable watching and listening to the crowd.

- For Step 3, you could then imagine being in a crowd where people brush against you and your child.

- Finally, in Step 4 you could combine all of these sensory elements.

As Another Example, if Your Child Resists Physical Affection...

- As Step 1, you could have your child imagine or remember being touched.

- In Step 2, if s/he is willing, you can touch a small spot on her or his body. For instance, your fingertip could touch the top of his/her hand (let your child specify what and where it's okay to touch.).

- For Step 3, you could touch his/her hand with your whole hand (or a few fingers—again, let your child set the parameters s/he is comfortable with).

- Finally, in Step 4 you could combine all of these sensory elements.

This exercise may be completed all at once or over a longer period of time. In the meantime, keep Tapping with your child whenever s/he is willing.

Chapter 10

"Negative" Emotions and How to Release Them

TAPPING WITH YOUR CHILD: ANGER

Anger is such a big, primal emotion that even as adults, it can feel like more than we can handle. We get so angry, it's "blinding"; so enraged, we're "boiling." Anger, and its unwieldy cousin rage, are such "hot" and overpowering emotions that we may try to suppress them, only to watch helplessly as they erupt at a later date. Or conversely, we may abandon the effort to control our anger and instead resort to frequent outbursts—which often leave us feeling angry all the time, inflicting even more damage on our relationships.

Not surprisingly, the simple act of allowing ourselves to feel and express anger feels taboo.

Yet anger is an unavoidable part of being human, as well as an essential defense mechanism.

*Studies also show that by repressing anger, we may be
increasing our risk of chronic pain, fibromyalgia and even
cancer, among other health issues.*[1]

So how can we release our anger in healthy ways, and through that process, teach our children how to express theirs similarly?

Sweet Relief (Minus the Mayhem)

Given that we rarely tolerate anger in ourselves, it can be especially hard to accept it from our children. Before we can help them learn to handle their anger better, let's first look at how we manage our own.

To begin, take a moment to think about your initial default reaction to anger. When you feel angry, do you tend hold it in or immediately let it all out?

If you tend to contain your anger, take a few minutes to do this next Tapping exercise on allowing yourself to feel and release your anger. After that, we'll do a second exercise on quieting the urge to unleash anger in potentially destructive ways.

Adult Tapping: Releasing the Taboo

One of the biggest obstacles to releasing anger is the hesitation so many of us experience around feeling and expressing it. But the bottom line is that if you don't let yourself feel anger, you can't release it.

That's where Tapping is so powerful, giving you a way to express and release your anger in a healthy way that will help you and support your relationships.

To begin, think back to a time when you felt angry but wouldn't let yourself express it. It doesn't matter why you were angry or whom you were mad at. No matter how big or small the event may be—it could be anger caused by a traffic jam or a huge fight with a loved one—focus on *one* time when you felt angry but couldn't express it.

On a scale of 0 to 10, how resistant did you feel about feeling and expressing your anger?

To begin, take 3 deep breaths. Start by Tapping 3 times on the Karate Chop point:

Karate Chop *(Repeat 3 times)*: Even though I don't think I can let myself feel this anger, I love myself and accept how I feel.

Eyebrow: This anger

Side of Eye: It doesn't feel safe

Under Eye: All this anger

Under Nose: I can't let myself feel it

Under Mouth: All this anger inside me

Collarbone: It's not safe to feel it

Under Arm: This anger scares me

Top of Head: It's so big, so hot

Eyebrow: I don't know how to handle it

Side of Eye: It doesn't seem to go away

Under Eye: I feel it in my body

Under Nose: This anger inside me

Under Mouth: Maybe I can let myself feel it

Collarbone: It's a part of me

Under Arm: And it's safe to feel it

Top of Head: Letting myself feel this anger now

Eyebrow: It's safe to feel this anger

Side of Eye: And it's safe to let it go

Under Eye: Letting myself feel it now

Under Nose: And letting it go

Under Mouth: I can feel this anger

Collarbone: And I can release it

Under Arm: Allowing myself to feel it

Top of Head: And let it go

Take a deep breath. On a scale of 0 to 10, how much resistance do you feel about feeling and expressing your anger now? Keep Tapping until you get the relief you desire.

Once you are more willing to feel your anger, you're ready to move on to the next exercise, which focuses on using Tapping to release your anger fully.

Adult Tapping: From Release to Peace

Since the most powerful way to use Tapping is in the moment when something is happening, begin by thinking about that same event that made you angry. Try to fill in the details of what made you so angry and why. As you recall it this time, let yourself feel your anger. Really open the mental floodgates and let your full anger rush out.

On a scale of 0 to 10, how intense is your anger? Give it a number now.

Begin by Tapping 3 times on the Karate Chop point, and proceed through all of the points for as many rounds as necessary.

While Tapping, imagine whatever or whomever you're angry at in front of you.

Either out loud or in your head, say what you'd say if you could vent everything you're feeling and thinking.

For example, let's say you're angry with your teenager for making you late to work again. Your Tapping might go something like this:

Eyebrow: I told you to get up!

Side of Eye: I can't be late to work again!

Under Eye: You have no idea how much stress this creates for me...

Under Nose: It makes me so mad that you don't even care...

Under Mouth: So angry right now!

Collarbone: You are so selfish...

Under Arm: You are so spoiled and it makes me furious!

Top of Head: I'm so angry right now, I could just lose it!

Keep Tapping, saying everything you need and want to say in the heat of the moment. It's important to let it all out, so if you finish and still feel angry, return to the exercise until you get the relief you desire.

When you're ready, take a deep breath, and check back in with your anger. How intense is it now on a scale of 0 to 10?

This is a powerful exercise to use anytime you're feeling angry. Return to it whenever and however often you need to.

Now that you've experienced a healthy way to release anger, let's look at how to tap with your children when they're angry.

Note: As always, when Tapping with your child, tailor your words to your child's age and experience.

Icky, Yucky Anger

This story is about Christine, a 6-year-old struggling with anger at her elementary school. Christine has been diagnosed with Autism Spectrum Disorder, but this story, along with the techniques her teacher uses, is powerful for all kids within a similar age range.

Christine was angry. Very angry. Earlier that day, her classmates had played the game she hates. It's called the "Zombie Game."

Since she often struggles with word recall and vocabulary, expressing her emotions is a challenge. Anger, in particular, often gets stuck inside her. Once that happens, she tends to become oppositional across the board, rejecting guidance and suggestions from peers, teachers and counselors alike.

Although Christine had done some Tapping previously, both in and out of class, she isn't always willing to tap when asked to by a teacher or counselor. This time when asked how angry she felt about the kids playing "The Zombie

Game," on a scale of 0 to 10 she said that her anger was an 11. She also shared that she didn't feel anger anywhere in her body. Committed to her oppositional stance, she then declined the chance to tap on her anger.

Hoping to find a way around Christine's opposition, her teacher suggested that she decorate a box to hold her anger. A talented artist who also loves to be read to, Christine agreed to do the project. This exercise is part of "The Box" technique, which can be used to contain issues that a child isn't ready to face, or when there isn't enough time to work through an issue. (See page 104 for more details about "The Box" technique.) The idea is to create a box that can contain emotions, memories and experiences until there is sufficient time and willingness to process and release them.

Although the box the child creates can be imaginary or real, for Christine, the experience of decorating her own box allowed her to shift her attention to something she loves to do, rather than focusing on her anger and opposition. She chose to draw hearts with pink and blue crayons on the box.

Once she had finished, the teacher wrote out her issue on an index card: "I am angry at an 11 about the Zombie Game." Christine and her teacher then placed the card inside the decorated box, and agreed to look back inside the box tomorrow. Once the index card was placed in the box, Christine seemed satisfied.

The next day, her teacher asked her if she'd be willing to look inside the box. As we saw in Chapter 9, asking a child's permission to look at an issue or emotion is incredibly important. In order to earn their trust and respect their boundaries, it's critical to request their permission to tap on something. Even when we know Tapping would really help at that moment, if a child isn't willing to try it, it's important to leave the box closed and wait until a time when they do feel ready.

In this case, Christine happily retrieved her box and opened it with the teacher. The teacher then read the card and asked if she felt ready to tap on her anger about the Zombie Game. Christine said no, so the teacher put the card back in the box.

Hoping to provide Christine with another protective distancing strategy, the teacher then read Christine a book about a girl who learns to express and release her anger. The book provided several opportunities to discuss anger and how the book's main character is feeling. Christine seemed to identify with the character, noting that the character's anger is also an 11 out of 10. By the end of the story, Christine said that the character's anger was now a 5 out of 10. They then discussed how the character handled her anger.

While discussing the book, the teacher asked Christine again if she felt willing to tap on her anger about the Zombie Game now. She agreed this time, but on one condition. She wanted the option to put her anger back in the box if she felt the need to. The teacher agreed, and they began Tapping.

Within a few rounds of Tapping, Christine's anger dissipated. She shared that her anger had gone down to a 0 out of 10. When the teacher asked how she knew that her anger was a 0, Christine answered, "I can play my own game." She then asked to sing the "Yicky Yucky" song, which the class usually sang together before the morning Tapping circle. She sang the song while Tapping through the points, seeming calm and happy.

The following week, a similar event happened where the kids excluded her from a game. Her reaction was significantly less intense, which allowed her to continue with her own play. That's great progress!

In spite of her results, Christine often continues to be oppositional, replying "no" when asked if she would like to tap. At random points throughout each day, though, she frequently taps on her own.

Given how much success Christine has had with Tapping, the teacher has allowed her to tap when she wants to. Even during morning circle, when the entire class taps together, Christine is allowed to join in or opt out. Since she's never forced to do her Tapping, she continues to tap on herself at random points during the school day.

Your Takeaways...

Here are a few valuable takeaways from Christine's story that apply to younger children who are angry, whether or not they have special needs:

- Christine's teacher went out of her way to meet Christine where she was. She never tried to force Tapping on her, and as a result, fostered trust.

- Her teacher personalized the experience by using Christine's enjoyment of art and books to get her more comfortable with using Tapping to release her anger.

- By introducing book characters that Christine could relate to, her teacher created a sense of comfort that allowed Christine to process and release her anger through Tapping. Especially with big, intense emotions like anger, using a "buffer" like this can be especially important.

Child Tapping: Releasing Anger (Younger Children)

Once you've introduced your child to Tapping and obtained his/her permission to try it with them on the anger they're feeling, try to get them to rate the intensity of that anger, either through the number scale (0 to 10) or using the "this much" method of measurement.

When possible, ask them where in their body they feel the anger, and how it feels. Also try to get a sense of what made them mad. If you get answers, use their words as often as you can.

Let's start Tapping!

Karate Chop *(Repeat 3 times)*: Even though I feel so mad, I'm a great kid and I'm okay.

Eyebrow: So mad!

Side of Eye: So mad right now!

Under Eye: So much anger

Under Nose: This yucky anger

Under Mouth: Don't like this yucky anger

Collarbone: It's okay to feel mad

Under Arm: All this icky, yucky anger

Top of Head: So much icky anger

Eyebrow: Maybe I can stop feeling this icky anger

Side of Eye: Letting it all go

Under Eye: I can feel quiet inside

Under Nose: I can smile inside

Under Mouth: No more icky anger

Collarbone: Letting it go now

Under Arm: Feeling quiet inside

Top of Head: Feeling smiley inside now

Check in with your child on their anger now. Continue Tapping until they get the desired relief.

If you can, slip in one round of positive Tapping to finish:

Eyebrow: I can feel smiley inside!

Side of Eye: I'm an awesome kid!

Under Eye: I can feel quiet inside now

Under Nose: I'm a great kid!

Under Mouth: It's okay to feel mad sometimes

Collarbone: I can tap on my magic points and feel better

Under Arm: I'm an awesome kid!

Top of Head: I can feel smiley inside whenever I want to!

Congratulations! If you've successfully led a younger child through 3 full rounds of Tapping, give yourself *and* them a huge hug. You've earned it! ☺

RELEASING ANGER TOWARD SIBLING(S)

Although fun at times, being a brother or sister isn't always easy. I can completely relate to stories like this one, shared recently by a mother of two. I'm sure my parents, like Loren's mom, would have appreciated knowing about Tapping back when my sister, my brother and I were irritating one another during most of our waking hours!

Loren, 9 years old, often got angry and frustrated with her 6-year-old sister, Alison. As she put it, she often felt "puffed up" when Alison wanted to talk or play with her. The worst, Loren added, was when Alison wanted to come into her room.

Talking to her mother about it one day, Loren explained that she felt like she had to play "mom" with Alison. She didn't like that role and often became angry when she felt pressured to play that part.

Wanting to help her enjoy Alison's company more, Loren's mom led her through several rounds of Tapping on releasing the responsibility of playing "mom" to Alison. They ended with a couple of rounds of Tapping on allowing herself to have more fun when Alison was around.

Once they were done Tapping, Loren felt much better. Ever since, she's had a much easier time accepting and appreciating her younger sister.

I love how Tapping helped Loren to voice her true feelings about not wanting to "play mommy" to her sister. By airing these emotions, Loren may be better able to foster a healthy, respectful relationship with Alison without the burden of unwanted responsibility.

Child Tapping: Releasing Anger toward Sibling(s)

First, let your child know they can safely share how they're feeling, and give them space to do so without judgment or comments. Once they've talked to you about how they're feeling, have them rate the intensity on a scale of 0 to 10 or using the "this much" method of measurement.

Take a deep breath, and begin by Tapping 3 times on the Karate Chop point.

Karate Chop (*Repeat 3 times*): Even though I'm so frustrated and annoyed with my brother/sister, I'm a great kid and it's okay to feel this way.

Eyebrow: I get so mad at him/her sometimes

Side of Eye: They bother me

Under Eye: They take my stuff

Under Nose: And come in my room

Under Mouth: I don't like it!

Collarbone: It makes me so mad

Under Arm: It's so frustrating!

Top of Head: Sometimes I just need to be alone

Eyebrow: Sometimes I just need to be with my friends

Side of Eye: It's okay to feel this way

Under Eye: I'm a great kid

Under Nose: And it's okay for me to feel these things

Under Mouth: I can let it go, too

Collarbone: I can spend time alone

Under Arm: And spend time just with my friends

Top of Head: Maybe then I can have more fun with my sibling

Eyebrow: I can let go of feeling mad

Side of Eye: And let go of feeling annoyed and frustrated with them

Under Eye: They just want to play with me

Under Nose: And spend time with me

Under Mouth: Maybe we can have more fun together, too

Collarbone: I'd like that!

Under Arm: I'm a great kid!

Top of Head: And I'm okay

Take a deep breath. Have your child rate their emotion(s) again. Keep Tapping until they get the desired relief.

Tough Exterior, Tender Heart

This story is about Gloria, a high school student from a broken home who struggles with anger at school. Like many children her age, Gloria's tough exterior hides her tender heart.

Enrolled in 10th grade in an inner-city high school, Gloria had been a chronically low achiever and consistent rule-breaker. Often rude with other students as well as superiors, she was notoriously hard to communicate with, and very concerned with what was (and wasn't) "cool."

Due to her numerous absences, as well as her refusal to complete assignments in and out of class, she was getting increasingly behind in her work. It was looking more and more like she wouldn't be able to graduate on time.

Concerned about Gloria's future, Steve, the school counselor, took her out of class one day to talk about how she could get back on track. While Gloria rarely shared details about her life out of school, he was fairly sure that she had little, if any, support at home. Steve wanted to do whatever he could to guide her.

Before he could finish his first sentence, Gloria began ranting about how her teacher had disrespected her. She was so angry that she couldn't even listen to what Steve was saying.

Steve, who'd been using Tapping for the past few years, asked Gloria if she'd be willing to try it. She was resistant at first, but then agreed. "She was humoring me," Steve explained. Since her willingness was all that Steve needed, he ignored her smirk and began Tapping.

Starting out, Gloria's anger was at a 7 out of 10. As they stood together in the hallway, he led Gloria through a few rounds of Tapping on her anger at her teacher. After only a few minutes of Tapping, her anger went down to a 3 out of 10.

The shift in Gloria's mood, body language and energy was striking. Within a few short minutes, her demeanor had changed completely. Obviously surprised herself, Gloria looked at Steve and shrugged. "That was weird," she commented.

"It was a memorable moment," Steve added as he recalled that day. "There are limits to what I can do for these kids, but the few minutes of Tapping we did that day clearly mattered. There was a very real shift that we both noticed."

In situations like these, we often focus on all of the unmet needs of a kid like Gloria. It *is* heartbreaking, and also incredibly unfair that kids should have to suffer in these ways. However, a single experience, like the shift Gloria experienced from Tapping, can plant a seed. Those few minutes of Tapping, however brief, *did* have a noticeable impact on Gloria. Her comment—"that was weird"—was her way of acknowledging the shift that she and Steve both clearly noticed.

Thanks to that one moment, she may realize that she can work with her brain to let go of her intense and overpowering emotions. That knowledge alone may eventually transform her relationship with her emotions, school, teachers, friends, even her entire life.

Before we look at how to tap on anger in situations like Gloria's, let's look at another similar story.

Managing Angry Outbursts

This story, shared by a high school counselor, is another great example of how useful Tapping is for releasing our most "explosive" emotions.

Isani had been in the foster system for several years. Angry with his mother, and suffering from neglect at home, even small provocations tended to throw him into a rage. On this particular day the school counselor had been called because Isani's outbursts were disrupting his 12th grade classroom.

After several minutes spent convincing Isani that he had to come to the counselor's office to talk, they both sat down. As soon as the counselor asked what had happened, Isani exploded.

Yelling as he told the story, he explained that a classmate had insulted him, and he'd had enough. To make matters worse, he hadn't slept the night before because something had happened to his grandmother.

As soon as he paused to take a breath, the counselor asked Isani if he'd be willing to do some Tapping. He nodded slightly. Like Gloria, he was skeptical, but also willing to try it. Since the counselor couldn't address the numerous issues Isani was facing outside of school, she focused their Tapping on his anger toward the classmate who had triggered him that day.

Within moments, Isani's anger went from a 10 out of 10 down to a 2 out of 10. The difference in his demeanor was remarkable. Suddenly calm and focused, he recalled the insult from his classmate and shrugged. The emotional charge was so minimal, it barely even registered.

Several weeks later, Isani told the school counselor that he'd been Tapping at night before bed. He was sleeping much more soundly than he had in years, and it was helping him to manage his anger also.

Considering how much adversity Isani had been facing, it's incredible that he's been able to improve his sleep, thanks to Tapping! The physical and emotional wellness benefits of improved sleep alone are enough to change his life. Just as important, he now understands that he has the power to transform his emotions and experiences. That knowledge alone can and will change his life forever.

Child Tapping: Releasing Anger (Middle School & High School Ages)

Children in middle- and high school often cling to rebellion. When, in addition to social pressure and the many other changes they're navigating, they're also facing challenges at home, the best thing you as a parent, teacher or counselor can do is to give them an experience of Tapping. For Gloria, that first experience of Tapping may be a seed that won't sprout for years; for Isani that single experience quickly became a way to self-regulate on a daily basis.

Your Takeaways...

- Tapping is especially powerful in the heat of the moment, when anger (or another emotion) is at its peak. If that's not possible, ask your child to recall a time when they felt angry.
- Once again, use their words whenever you can.
- If/when they're willing, let them do the talking while they tap.

- Avoid power struggles by respecting their boundaries, even when that means not Tapping at a time when they may need to.

Child Tapping: Quieting an Angry Outburst

Let's do some Tapping on helping your child to release anger when it arises.

To begin, have him or her rate the intensity of his/her anger on a scale of 0 to 10.

If you can, ask them to take a deep breath. Then begin Tapping:

Karate Chop *(Repeat 3 times)*: Even though I feel all this anger boiling inside me, I'm great and I accept how I feel.

Eyebrow: So much anger

Side of Eye: All this anger inside me

Under Eye: I can feel it in my body

Under Nose: So much anger in me

Under Mouth: It feels bigger than me

Collarbone: Like an explosion that's about to go off

Under Arm: So much anger in me

Top of Head: I can feel it now

Eyebrow: This big, hot anger in me

Side of Eye: I can feel it in my body now

Under Eye: Feeling this anger now

Under Nose: And letting it go

Under Mouth: Letting myself feel it now

Collarbone: And then letting it go

Under Arm: I can release this anger now

Top of Head: And allow myself to feel calm inside

Eyebrow: I can feel quiet and calm now

Side of Eye: Releasing any leftover anger now

Under Eye: Feeling calm and quiet inside

Under Nose: Feeling calm in my body

Under Mouth: And quiet in my mind

Collarbone: Letting any remaining anger go now

Under Arm: Allowing myself to relax

Top of Head: Feeling peaceful in mind and body now

Ask your child to rate his/her anger now on a scale of 0 to 10. Keep Tapping on his/her anger, and any other related issues that came up while Tapping, for as long as s/he is willing, or until s/he gets the desired relief.

TAPPING WITH YOUR CHILD: FEARS AND PHOBIAS

In Chapter 2 we looked at the *stress response*, also known as the *fight-or-flight response*. That mind-body process, which is intimately connected to our survival instinct, demonstrates how hard-wired we are to feel fear. And so it is not surprising that, as children and as adults, fear is an emotion with which we're constantly engaging, whether by feeling it or resisting it.

Before we begin looking at how to use Tapping with children on their fears, let's do some Tapping on any fear that you may be feeling. By having your own experience Tapping on a fear, you'll feel more comfortable using it with your child.

Adult Tapping: Releasing Fear

What most often causes you to feel fear? Are you afraid your child won't be willing to try Tapping? Are you often afraid of being late to work and other appointments? Do you fear confrontation or not being able to fall asleep at night?

However big or small, pick something that makes you feel afraid. If you feel that fear in your body, notice where in your body you feel it and also how it feels.

Next, rate the intensity of your fear on a scale of 0 to 10.

Let's begin by Tapping 3 times on the Karate Chop point:

Karate Chop *(Repeat 3 times)*: Even though I feel all this fear in my body, I love myself and accept how I feel.

Eyebrow: All this fear

Side of Eye: So much fear in my body

Under Eye: This fear has a grip on me

Under Nose: All this fear

Under Mouth: It's got a hold on me

Collarbone: I can feel it in my body

Under Arm: So much fear

Top of Head: It's safe to feel it now

Eyebrow: I can feel this fear now

Side of Eye: And I can let it go

Under Eye: It's safe to feel this fear

Under Nose: And it's safe to let it go

Under Mouth: I don't need this fear to be safe

Collarbone: I can let it go now

Under Arm: It's safe to release this fear

Top of Head: It's safe to feel safe

Eyebrow: Letting any remaining fear go now

Side of Eye: Releasing from my mind and body

Under Eye: I don't need this fear anymore

Under Nose: I'm letting it go

Under Mouth: It's safe to let go of this fear

Collarbone: And it's safe to feel safe

Under Arm: Feeling relaxed and calm now

Top of Head: It's safe to feel safe now

Take a deep breath and give your fear a number of intensity on a scale of 0 to 10. Keep Tapping until you get the desired relief.

Now that you've had an experience with Tapping on fear, let's look at stories about how to use Tapping with your child when s/he is feeling afraid.

Fear of Swallowing Medicine

When she was diagnosed with ADHD, Francesca, 12 years old, was instructed by her doctor to take daily medication to moderate her symptoms. Immediately, however, she refused to take her daily pill. A few days into her refusals, she admitted to her mom that she was afraid of choking while swallowing the pill.

When her mom asked her if she'd be willing to tap on her fear of choking on the pill, Francesca agreed. As they began to tap, they remembered a time when, at 2 years old, she'd begun choking on a hard caramel candy that someone had given her. Her mom had had to slap her back and turn her upside down to get the candy out of her throat. Although she'd quickly moved on, it was clear the memory still haunted her.

Francesca's mother led her through Tapping to neutralize the emotional charge of that traumatic event. The next day Francesca took her medication willingly, and since then, she's been able to take even larger pills without issue.

I share this story not to endorse any particular treatment for ADHD. While I'm obviously a fan of Tapping, each case is unique, and needs to be treated as such. To me this story is simply a great example of how Tapping can help children overcome their fears.

Child Tapping: Overcoming Fears Related to Past Events

When a current fear or phobia is related to a past event, it's often necessary to neutralize the emotional intensity of that original event by Tapping on it. First, though, it's best to "test the waters," so to speak, by Tapping on the current fear. For Francesca, that would look something like this:

Karate Chop *(Repeat 3 times)*: Even though I'm so afraid of swallowing this pill every morning, I'm a great kid and everything's okay.

Eyebrow: So scared of swallowing this pill

Side of Eye: I'll choke if I try it

Under Eye: I can't swallow this pill

Under Nose: So scared I'll choke

Under Mouth: It's okay that I feel scared

Collarbone: My mom would never let me choke

Under Arm: It's safe to let this fear go now

Top of Head: I'm safe even when I'm swallowing a pill

Tap through a few rounds and then have your child rate his/her fear again.

If Tapping on the current fear doesn't provide sufficient relief, you may then need to tap on the original trigger event. When that's the case, especially with younger kids, stick to Tapping on the fear s/he felt during the original event, rather than describing the event in graphic detail. As soon as you see a shift in her/his mood, move on to the positive. For Francesca, Tapping on the original trigger event might look like this:

Eyebrow: I was so scared

Side of Eye: I couldn't breathe

Under Eye: It was so scary

Under Nose: I couldn't breathe

Under Mouth: I was so afraid

Collarbone: My mom was there

Under Arm: And she cleared my throat

Top of Head: I could breathe right away after that

Eyebrow: That candy was too big for me

Side of Eye: I was only 2 years old

Under Eye: I was too little for that candy

Under Nose: I'm bigger now

Under Mouth: And my mom's right here

Collarbone: It's a little pill

Under Arm: I can swallow it easily now

Top of Head: I won't choke on this pill

Eyebrow: My mom's right here with me

Side of Eye: I'm safe

Under Eye: I can swallow this pill easily now!

Under Nose: I'm safe and I don't need to be scared anymore

Under Mouth: I can do this!

Collarbone: I'm an awesome kid!

Under Arm: My mom's here and I'm safe

Top of Head: I'm a great kid and I can do this!

Take a deep breath. Check back in on the intensity of your child's fear, and keep Tapping until s/he gets the desired relief. Once you've checked in on the current moment, then it may be time to tap on the original traumatic event.

Releasing the Fear of Needles

Laurel, 6 years old, became visibly terrified when her doctor requested a blood test. She broke down in tears and clutched her doll tightly to her chest. The pediatric nurse, who had used Tapping with her child patients for years, first suggested that they apply topical numbing cream to her arm to prevent the ouchies. Laurel immediately shook her head no, and held her arms tightly to her chest.

Noticing the intensity of Laurel's fear, the nurse suggested that they play a game. They practiced Tapping gently on the nearby desk to make a "bonking noise." Then they began Tapping through the points on the body as the nurse voiced Laurel's fears about needles as well as the numbing cream.

When they were done Tapping, the nurse asked if she could put numbing cream on Laurel's doll. Laurel agreed, and helped to apply the bandage to her doll once the numbing cream had been applied.

Without any resistance or hesitation, Laurel then consented to have numbing cream applied to both of her arms. About 20 minutes later, once the numbing cream had taken effect, Laurel had her blood taken without any upset. Her mother was amazed and relieved by the transformation.

Most children are afraid of needles, and in some cases those fears turn into phobias. By respecting Laurel's emotions and boundaries while also addressing her fear at a moment of peak intensity, the nurse was able to achieve great results.

Let's look at how you can tap with your child on their fear of needles.

Child Tapping: **Overcoming the Fear of Needles**

First have your child rate their fear of needless on a scale of 0 to 10 or using the "this much" method of measurement.

The following script is based on the Tapping exercise the pediatric nurse used with Laurel, but as always, change words and phrasing to match your child's experience.

Take a deep breath, and begin by Tapping 3 times on the Karate Chop point:

Karate Chop (*Repeat 3 times*): Even though I am afraid of having a blood test, I love myself and I'm a great kid.

Eyebrow: I'm really scared to have this blood test

Side of Eye: It's going to hurt

Under Eye: The needle is really sharp and scary

Under Nose: I don't like having blood tests

Under Mouth: I'm scared to let them take my blood

Collarbone: I'm scared it's going to hurt

Under Arm: I can't do this

Top of Head: I'm scared to have this blood test

Eyebrow: What if it won't hurt as bad as I think?

Side of Eye: What if the numbing cream helps to prevent the ouch

Under Eye: I might be okay if I use the numbing cream

Under Nose: I won't be alone

Under Mouth: My doll will be with me

Collarbone: Maybe my doll will get the numbing cream too

Under Arm: The numbing cream will help so I don't feel the needle poke

Top of Head: They need to see my blood

Eyebrow: This is to keep me healthy

Side of Eye: I might see my blood if I look

Under Eye: I won't even feel it

Under Nose: I'll feel the squishy rubber band on my arm

Under Mouth: It will feel tight but I'll be okay

Collarbone: They're very good at taking kids' blood

Under Arm: They take blood from tiny little babies

Top of Head: I'll be okay when they take my blood

Take a deep breath, and ask your child to measure the intensity of his/her fear now. Keep Tapping until s/he gets the desired relief.

Releasing the Fear of Spiders

Marla's fear of spiders had grown more intense the older she got. It had become an obstacle to her sense of safety as well, given that she lived with her family in a warm climate where spiders were prevalent year-round.

Hoping to help her overcome her fear, her mother asked her if she'd be willing to do some Tapping to make her fear of spiders go away. She nodded silently. Her mother then led her through a few rounds of Tapping, using words and phrases she'd heard her daughter use. They tapped on spiders being ugly, disgusting and scary. They tapped on how seeing a spider made a creepy, tingling feeling go down her spine. They also tapped on the fact that thinking about spiders sometimes kept her awake at night.

Within a few rounds of Tapping, Marla's fear went from a 10 out of 10 down to a 2. She then asked her mother if they could stop Tapping. She explained that she didn't want all of her fear to go away, because then she might lose all of her fear and play with spiders.

Child Tapping: Releasing the Fear of Spiders (And Other Creatures)

Below is a sample Tapping script for fear of spiders in younger children. Feel free to adapt it for other fears—fear of snakes, bees, etc. by changing the words.

Start by measuring the intensity of their fear, either on a scale of 0 to 10 or using the "this much" method of measurement. Then start by Tapping 3 times on the Karate Chop point:

Karate Chop *(Repeat 3 times)*: Even though I'm so scared of those icky, creepy spiders, I'm a great kid and I'm okay!

Eyebrow: So scared of the creepy spiders

Side of Eye: Those icky spiders

Under Eye: They scare me

Under Nose: They come out of nowhere

Under Mouth: So scared of the creepy spiders

Collarbone: So scary

Under Arm: Don't like the creepy, icky spiders

Top of Head: That's okay

Eyebrow: I'm much bigger than those creepy spiders

Side of Eye: I'm safe

Under Eye: They scare me

Under Nose: But I'm okay

Under Mouth: I can say bye-bye to being scared

Collarbone: I can feel quiet inside now

Under Arm: Even when I see creepy spiders

Top of Head: Even when I think about creepy spiders

Eyebrow: Saying bye-bye to being scared

Side of Eye: I'm safe

Under Eye: I don't have to be scared anymore

Under Nose: I can feel quiet inside

Under Mouth: Even when I see spiders

Collarbone: I'm safe

Under Arm: I'm an awesome kid!

Top of Head: I'm okay!

Take another deep breath, and ask your child to measure the intensity of his/her fear now. Keep Tapping until s/he gets the desired relief.

If there was a trigger event for his/her fear, and it seems necessary to tap through that, keep it simple and use what *s/he* remembers. For instance, depending on the event, your Tapping might look something like:

"That time it crawled on my arm"

"That creepy spider was right in front of my face"

"I almost stepped on that snake"

"That time a bee stung me"

"That time I got a spider bite"

Tap through your child's memories until the emotional intensity is cleared. You may need to tap through more than once, which is normal, so keep Tapping with your child whenever s/he is open to it.

Child Tapping: Releasing the Resistance to Completely Eliminate a Fear

Looking back at Marla's story about her fear of spiders, while she made huge progress with Tapping, she also made a point of stopping her Tapping before she'd eliminated her fear altogether. Instead, she explained, she needed to keep some of her fear to prevent her from getting so comfortable with spiders that she began playing with them.

As sweet as her reasoning is, this attachment to her own fear is actually another great Tapping target. She may be holding onto a limiting belief that she needs fear to protect her. That belief may become a limitation later on in life.

If you notice similar resistance in your child around eliminating his/her fear(s), try suggesting that you tap together on that resistance. In Marla's case, that Tapping might look something like this:

Karate Chop *(Repeat 3 times)*: Even though I'm afraid of Tapping away my fear completely, I'm a great kid and I'm okay.

Eyebrow: I'm scared to let go of this fear all the way

Side of Eye: I need this fear to keep me safe

Under Eye: What if I start playing with spiders?

Under Nose: I need this fear

Under Mouth: I can't trust myself without this fear

Collarbone: I might start playing with spiders

Under Arm: I need this fear to keep me safe

Top of Head: Why do I need this fear to keep me safe?

Eyebrow: I don't have to play with spiders

Side of Eye: And I don't have to hold onto this fear, either

Under Eye: I'm safe on my own

Under Nose: I don't need this fear to keep me safe

Under Mouth: I'm safe without this fear

Collarbone: I don't need this fear

Under Arm: I'm already safe

Top of Head: It's safe to let go of this fear

Eyebrow: I don't need it anymore

Side of Eye: I'm safe on my own

Under Eye: And I'll be safe around spiders

Under Nose: I don't need fear

Under Mouth: I know not to play with spiders

Collarbone: I'm safe without this fear

Under Arm: I'm safe feeling safe

Top of Head: I can feel relaxed and safe when I let go of the remainder of this fear

Check back in with your child on how resistant s/he feels now about letting his/her fear/phobia go. Keep Tapping until s/he no longer feels resistance around releasing the remainder of his/her fear. When s/he is ready, do some Tapping on releasing that last part of the original fear or phobia.

Fear of Swimming—Sharks & Crocodiles

Kyle didn't want to go to his swimming lessons. Water was too dangerous, he said, since it's where sharks and crocodiles live. He had seen footage on television of a great white shark attacking a surfer. He'd also seen footage of crocodiles jumping at people on land and in small boats.

At 6 years old, Kyle had developed a fairly intense phobia of water. Meeting with an EFT practitioner, Deirdre, for the second time, Kyle began to share what he had seen on television. Deirdre then asked him to draw the shark and the crocodile that he'd seen. When he was done with his drawing, she told him he could rip up the drawing. He did so, and seemed to gain some satisfaction from the exercise.

She then asked him how he felt about swimming in the pool. He said he still felt like a bit of a scaredy cat. They did several rounds of Tapping on feeling like a scaredy cat. As they tapped, Deirdre used setup statements like:

"Even though I'm a bit of a scaredy cat in the pool because of the shark and crocodile, I'm a great and happy kid and I'm stronger than anybody else and stronger than a shark and a crocodile."

By the end of their Tapping, Kyle said that he felt "fine."

During a Tapping session a week or two later, Kyle shared that he'd had a dream about a shark. In the dream he and the shark kept swapping teeth. Finally, Kyle got the bigger set of teeth and he bit the shark. Although the dream may sound harsh, dreams like this one can be an indication that the dreamer is taking his or her power back, since he/she is no longer a victim.

During a separate session, Kyle talked about going to swimming lessons. He shared that he is still a bit scared when he swims in one specific pool where he can't see the edge. Rather than avoiding the water, however, he learned to move out of the way when he thought a shark was coming so the shark would just run into the wall.

As we've already seen, especially with younger children, it can be helpful to skip the 0 to 10 SUD scale. Instead, go with the flow and use their language, even when it initially seems overly vague and/or nonsensical.

Before we do a Tapping exercise on this issue, let's look at one more story on a related topic.

Fear of Water

It had been years since Rebecca had become terrified of water. Now 9 years old, she was also becoming increasingly annoyed with her fear. She wanted to swim with her friends. She wanted to feel as happy and carefree as they seemed to be in the water.

When asked why she was afraid of water, Rebecca explained that she'd loved the water until the day that Anne, her older sister, had tried to drown her. Given that the event was still so vivid in Rebecca's mind, instead of Tapping on statements, her counselor asked her to tell the story while Tapping through the points. The counselor made sure to tap along with her so that Rebecca could easily follow along while focusing on her memories of that day.

While Tapping through the points, Rebecca recalled the moments when her sister had jokingly grabbed her from the shallow end of the pool and flung Rebecca into the deep end. Rebecca landed near the side of the pool, but still too far to grab the edge. Instead of grasping the side, she'd been completely immersed in the water. When Rebecca emerged from the water, Anne had a devious look on her face that made Rebecca think she'd purposely tried to drown her. Terrified and confused, Rebecca watched as her sister approached her as she flailed, petrified that she might drown. Anne then dragged Rebecca back to the shallow end of the pool. Although Rebecca was once again able to breathe, her fear of drowning still felt very real.

Continuing to tap through the points, Rebecca retold the story four times, each time adding more details. Without any interruption from the counselor, Rebecca continued to tap and talk through her memories. Her mood lightened considerably, and by the end of one hour of Tapping, Rebecca felt totally comfortable with the idea of swimming in the deep end of the pool. Two days later Rebecca joined a swim club.

Both Rebecca and Kyle's stories show how powerful Tapping is for overcoming fears and phobias. I love how they both used some form of visualization—Rebecca mentally "walked through" her memory, while Kyle had a powerful dream—to create a new relationship with water.

This story was graciously provided by:
http://www.eft-tapping.learnandenjoy.com/eft-children-fear-water.html

Child Tapping: **Overcoming Fear of Water**

First, let your child know you want them to tell the story of what they remember as they tap through the points. You can either tap on the points for them, or have them follow you as you tap along with them.

Begin by measuring the intensity of the fear, whether on a scale of 0 to 10 or using the "this much" method of measurement.

Take a deep breath together, and begin with the Eyebrow point as they tell the story. If they're open to it, have them pause at the scariest parts of the story to tap on those moments until the emotional intensity is gone.

For Rebecca, that might have meant pausing to do additional Tapping on two peak scary moments—when her sister threw her in the deep end, and when she saw the devious look on her sister's face and feared for her life. Let's see how that might look:

Let's say the intensity of Rebecca's general memory of the trigger event is an 8 out of 10, but it increases to a 10 out of 10 when she recalls those seconds when she was being thrown into the deep end. In that case, the adult Tapping with Rebecca could do the following:

- Gently ask her to pause the story at that point, and do several rounds of Tapping just on that moment until the intensity has gone down. She can then move ahead with telling her story while continuing to tap.

- She would then repeat that same process with the second peak intensity moment (when she saw the mischievous look in her sister's eye and feared for her life).

- When the emotional charge of that second peak moment has gone down, she'd then continue Tapping through the story.

- To test her results, Rebecca would ideally retell the story from start to finish, Tapping the whole time, until she could run through her entire memory without feeling afraid.

Especially with younger children, it can be hard to follow this entire process from start to finish. If interrupting the child's story causes them to feel unwilling to tap, don't worry about pausing to tap on peak moments. Instead, have them tell and retell the story until the emotional intensity is gone. As we've seen, when we're Tapping with kids, we may need to bend the so-called "rules" in order to get the best results.

Overcoming The Fear of a Scary Movie

At 6 years old, Steven had watched a movie at a friend's house that had scared him deeply. Although PG-rated, the movie had included several dark and scary scenes that remained vivid in his memory weeks later. His fear had grown so intense that even routine tasks like getting dressed and going to the bathroom had become an issue. Whenever scenes from the movie ran through his head, including in his nightmares, he would begin screaming and crying uncontrollably.

After several weeks had passed, his parents decided to try Tapping with him whenever he remembered the movie. Within several months of repeated Tapping through the movie scenes he was remembering, his fears went away, and he was no longer afraid to do simple, routine tasks, such as going to the bathroom, by himself.

Of all of the five senses, vision occupies the largest area of the human brain. Not surprisingly, scary images and scenes often have a lasting impact, especially on children. Whether it's a TV show, movie or even a scary commercial that you didn't intend your child to watch, Tapping is a powerful tool for helping children release their fears.

Child Tapping: **Releasing Fear(s) from a Scary Movie**

This is a time when it's particularly important to let your child lead the way as much as possible. Since fear easily overpowers rational thinking, try to resist the temptation to tell your child that the movie or character isn't real. Instead, focus your attention and Tapping on recreating a sense of safety, which is what will cause his/her fear to dissipate.

Limit your Tapping on the elements that scared him/her, and leave out other parts. For example, I have a friend whose child was scared by a huge robot he saw in a movie "because it was so big, it could crush people." In that case, your Tapping might go like this:

Start by asking your child to measure the intensity of his/her fear, either through the number scale, or using the "this much" method of measurement.

Then begin by Tapping 3 times on the Karate Chop point:

Karate Chop *(Repeat 3 times)*: Even though that scary robot is so big it could crush people, I'm a great kid and I'm okay!

Eyebrow: That scary robot

Side of Eye: So big

Under Eye: It can crush people

Under Nose: So scary

Under Mouth: I don't like that robot

Collarbone: It's too big

Under Arm: That big, scary robot

Top of Head: I don't like it

Eyebrow: I'm safe

Side of Eye: I'm a great kid!

Under Eye: And I'm safe

Under Nose: I don't like that big, scary robot

Under Mouth: But I'm a great kid

Collarbone: And I'm safe

Under Arm: I'm an awesome kid!

Top of Head: And I'm safe

Eyebrow: I'm a great kid

Side of Eye: That robot can't hurt me

Under Eye: I'm safe

Under Nose: That robot can't hurt me!

Under Mouth: I'm safe

Collarbone: I'm a great kid!

Under Arm: I don't have to be scared now

Top of Head: I'm an awesome kid, and I'm safe

Again, have your child measure the intensity of his/her fear of the scary movie. Keep Tapping until s/he gets the desired relief.

Releasing the Fear of Swings

Since children don't always vocalize how they're feeling, it can be challenging for parents and other supporting adults to figure out how different experiences and emotions are affecting one another. One of the many things I love about Tapping is how simply and directly it can resolve what seem like emotionally complex situations. This story is yet another great example of that.

For the past few years, Lara, 7 years old, had been afraid of swings. Although her parents had always hoped she'd outgrow her fear, it had grown more intense, especially once her parents began what quickly became a tumultuous divorce.

During a playdate one day at a friend's house, Lara's mom, Liz, sat on the swing in her backyard and invited Lara to sit in the swing alongside her. Reluctantly, Lara sat in the swing, which her mom steadied for her.

Liz assured Lara that she would hold her hand as they sat together on the swing set. She then asked Lara if she'd be willing to try a "cool new thing" called Tapping that might help her feel safer on swings. Lara nodded yes, and said that she was willing to try it as long as no one pushed the swing. Liz agreed not to push the swing without Lara's permission.

Her mom then began Tapping on Lara's Karate Chop point and asked her where in her body she felt the fear. She replied that it was in her tummy. Lara then began sharing her memories of times when she'd felt afraid on swings. Her mom continued Tapping gently on her, moving through the Tapping points as she listened.

Purely as the result of Lara's own natural body movements, the swing began to move. As they continued talking, Liz continued to tap through the points on Lara's body. The swing began to move faster, but Lara didn't seem to notice. A couple of minutes later, Lara and her friend jumped off of the swings to go and play a game.

From that point forward, Lara's fear of swings was a thing of the past. Whether on the swing in their backyard or at the playground, Lara would jump on and swing without hesitation.

Amazing! What a huge transformation, and one that may plant the seed for many more positive changes down the road.

Child Tapping: Eliminating Fears & Phobias ("Scan the Body" Technique)

Since children are often more attuned to the body than adults, pinpointing where they feel fears and phobias in the body can be especially powerful.

To begin, have your child answer questions like:

- Where in your body do you feel this fear/phobia?
- What does this fear/phobia feel like in your body—tight, hot/cold, tingly, buzzing, clenched, prickly, nervous, fluttering, icky, etc.?

Next have your child rate the intensity of the fear s/he feels in her/his body, either on a scale of 0 to 10 or using the "this much" method of measurement.

Then begin Tapping, focusing on the physical manifestations of his/her fear. For example, if your child feels sick to their stomach when they think about going on a rollercoaster ride, your Tapping might go like this:

Karate Chop *(Repeat 3 times)*: Even though my stomach feels sick when I think about riding on that rollercoaster, I'm an awesome kid and everything's okay!

Eyebrow: That scary rollercoaster ride

Side of Eye: I feel sick in my tummy when I think about it

Under Eye: I don't like that scary rollercoaster ride

Under Nose: It makes me feel sick

Under Mouth: That scary rollercoaster ride

Collarbone: It makes my tummy feel sick

Under Arm: That ride was so scary

Top of Head: But I'm okay!

Eyebrow: It scared me so badly

Side of Eye: But I'm okay

Under Eye: I'm an awesome kid

Under Nose: Everything's okay

Under Mouth: I'm safe

Collarbone: That rollercoaster ride really scared me

Under Arm: But I'm a great kid

Top of Head: And everything's okay

Eyebrow: I'm safe

Side of Eye: And everything's okay

Under Eye: I can feel calm now

Under Nose: I can let go of this scared feeling in my tummy

Under Mouth: I can feel calm

Collarbone: And know that I'm safe

Under Arm: I'm an awesome kid

Top of Head: I can feel safe and calm now

Have your child rate the intensity of the fear in his/her tummy now. Keep Tapping until s/he gets the desired relief.

Child Tapping: Eliminating the Fear of the Dark

If your child is afraid of the dark, begin by having him/her rate his/her fear on a 0 to 10 scale or using the "this much" method of measurement.

Take a deep breath. Start by Tapping 3 times on the Karate Chop point:

Karate Chop *(Repeat 3 times)*: Even though I get so scared in the dark, I'm a great kid and I'm okay.

Eyebrow: So scared of the dark

Side of Eye: I can't see anything

Under Eye: It's so scary

Under Nose: It's so dark

Under Mouth: I can't see anything

Collarbone: I get so scared

Under Arm: That's okay

Top of Head: I'm a great kid!

Eyebrow: Everything's okay

Side of Eye: I'm a great kid

Under Eye: And I'm safe

Under Nose: Even in the dark

Under Mouth: I'm safe

Collarbone: And everything's okay

Under Arm: Even when it's really dark

Top of Head: I'm safe

Eyebrow: I can feel calm now

Side of Eye: I can feel safe in the dark

Under Eye: I'm safe

Under Nose: I'm a great kid

Under Mouth: And I'm safe, even in the dark

Collarbone: I'm a great kid

Under Arm: And I can feel safe in the dark

Top of Head: I'm a great kid and I'm okay

When s/he is ready, have her/him rate her/his fear of the dark again.

If your child expresses fear of shadows or shapes s/he sees in the dark, have her/him tap through the points as s/he talks about what it looks like and what s/he is afraid of until that fear is gone.

With fears like this that a child inevitably faces on a routine basis, regular Tapping is especially important.

You can also gradually ease your child into being comfortable in the dark. If s/he is afraid of turning off their light at night, buy several night-lights for her/his room, and as s/he continues Tapping on her/his fear and getting more comfortable in the dark, you can try removing one night each week until s/he is sleeping with only one or two night-lights in the room.

Releasing Fear of Loud Noises & Sirens

Taylor, a 3rd grader, had a complete meltdown during a fire drill. Hoping to give her a tool that she could use herself, the school counselor, Emily, spoke with Taylor's mother about Tapping, and got her permission to try it with Taylor.

Having been previously diagnosed with ADD and Asperger's syndrome, Taylor had a long list of questions about Tapping. To begin the process while also respecting Taylor's need for answers, Emily asked her to tap on the Karate Chop point along with her while Taylor asked all of her questions.

Once Taylor was satisfied with the information Emily had given her, they continued Tapping on the Karate Chop point while Taylor told the story of her first fire drill. She was 4 years old and in preschool. The siren had terrified her, and she didn't understand what was happening, which made the event even scarier. Remembering that day, Taylor said that the emotional intensity she experienced was a 10 out of 10.

They then tapped two rounds of EFT using the following setup statement:

"Even though I can't stand the sound of the fire drill, I know I'm a good girl and I am willing to believe I'm safe."

As the emotional intensity of that memory lowered, they continued Tapping on the different elements of the event, including the unexpected loud noise, not knowing what was happening and wanting to be comforted.

As they continued Tapping, Taylor then visualized herself as that 4-year-old girl scared of the fire drill. While Tapping, she then comforted the 4-year-old girl she used to be, using reminder phrases like:

- I didn't know there was going to be a fire drill.

- I was so scared.

- I just wanted someone to help me or give me a hug,

- I was only 4 years old and didn't know what to do.

- Now I have some strategies.

- I'm almost 9 years old now.

- I was so scared when I was 4 years old.

By the end of their Tapping, Taylor's fear and anxiety had gone down to a 3 out of 10. "Now I know what to do to help myself if I'm scared," she said. Emily then gave her homework, which was to continue Tapping at home and on the car ride to school. Emily also gave her some Tapping statements to use if they felt comfortable.

Since that session, Taylor has successfully completed a fire drill. Immediately following the fire drill she tapped with Emily in order to process the event. By using Tapping on every relevant component of Taylor's fear, she's giving Taylor the chance to eliminate her fear faster and with greater ease.

Your Takeaway...

- Whenever possible, use Tapping to neutralize the original event, as well as relevant before/after current events that evoke your child's fear.

Child Tapping: Overcoming the Fear of Loud Noises (Sirens, Etc.)

To begin, have your child rate his/her fear of loud noises and/or sirens, either on a scale of 0 to 10 or using the "this much" method of measurement.

Start by Tapping 3 times on the Karate Chop point:

Karate Chop (*Repeat 3 times*): Even though I really don't like those loud noises, I'm an awesome kid and I'm okay!

Eyebrow: So many loud noises

Side of Eye: Too loud!

Under Eye: They hurt my ears

Under Nose: I don't like them

Under Mouth: They scare me

Collarbone: Those loud noises

Under Arm: So scary

Top of Head: I don't like them

Eyebrow: I don't like those loud noises

Side of Eye: They scare me

Under Eye: That's okay

Under Nose: I'm safe

Under Mouth: And I'm a great kid

Collarbone: I'm safe

Under Arm: Even when there are loud noises

Top of Head: I'm safe

Eyebrow: I'm a great kid

Side of Eye: I can feel safe when there are loud noises

Under Eye: They scare me sometimes

Under Nose: That's okay

Under Mouth: I'm safe!

Collarbone: I'm a great kid

Under Arm: And I'm okay

Top of Head: I can feel safe when there are loud noises

Take a deep breath. Ask your child to rate the intensity of his/her fear now, and keep Tapping until s/he gets the desired relief.

If your child's fear is still present, and/or you know it's connected to a past event, refer back to the "Tell the Story" technique on Page 103 of Chapter 8.

TAPPING WITH YOUR CHILD: SADNESS

Sadness is one of those emotions that can feel too big to handle. Although it can be intense, sadness is considered to be a healthy emotional response to events and circumstances. Unlike depression, which is characterized by emotional numbness, sadness can feel acute—so much so that, over time, we may begin to fear it.

On a cultural level, our fear of sadness often leads to statements like "Don't cry, you'll be okay." However well-intended these responses may be, when they are offered to children, particularly young children, they can be interpreted as instructions to avoid feeling sadness altogether.

When we consider how painful sadness is, this may seem to be a good thing. But the downside is that avoiding sadness is only possible when we limit our ability to feel all emotions, including joy, excitement and other healthy, positive feelings. As a result, by limiting how much sadness we feel, we're likely to experience less happiness rather than more.

As with all emotions, the best way to process sadness is by allowing it to be felt and then released. Using Tapping, your child can access his/her sadness on both a mental and physical level, which will allow for a quicker and more powerful release.

As always, the best place to start is with Tapping on your own stress and emotions. We'll do that first, and then look at how to use Tapping with your child to release his/her sadness.

Adult Tapping: **Making Peace with Sadness**

Do you let yourself feel sadness, or constantly try to avoid or disrupt it? To help your child learn to process and release his/her sadness, it's important to let go of your own feelings about sadness.

To begin, think of something that makes you feel sad, and notice how intensely you want to push that thought away and out of your mind. Rate the intensity of that urge on a scale of 0 to 10.

Take a deep breath, and begin by Tapping 3 times on the Karate Chop point.

Karate Chop *(Repeat 3 times)*: Even though I feel all this resistance around letting myself feel sadness, I deeply and completely love and accept myself.

Eyebrow: This sadness

Side of Eye: This deep, overwhelming sadness

Under Eye: I don't want to face it

Under Nose: I don't want to feel it

Under Mouth: I want to push it away

Collarbone: This sadness

Under Arm: I want to turn away from it

Top of Head: It's too big and overwhelming to feel

Eyebrow: This sadness

Side of Eye: It feels all-consuming

Under Eye: I want to push it away

Under Nose: I don't want my child to have to feel it, either

Under Mouth: It's too overwhelming

Collarbone: Maybe I can let myself feel it

Under Arm: Even though it hurts

Top of Head: I don't like feeling this sadness

Eyebrow: I don't want my child to feel sadness

Side of Eye: That's okay

Under Eye: It's not fun to feel sadness

Under Nose: It's safe to feel sadness

Under Mouth: I don't have to fear sadness

Collarbone: It's safe to let my child feel sadness

Under Arm: It's safe to feel safe with sadness

Top of Head: It's safe to feel safe with sadness

Take a deep breath, and check back in your willingness to feel sadness now. Has your resistance to feeling sadness decreased? Keep Tapping until you get the desired relief.

Now that you've had an experience, let's look at how you can use Tapping with your child to help him/her release sadness.

Note: As always, when Tapping with your child, tailor your words to your child's age and experience.

WHAT'S YOUR CHILD'S SADNESS ABOUT?

Sadness is an emotion we feel *about* something. However for a child, the reason for feeling sadness may not always be clear. If your child is feeling sad but isn't yet clear on what that sadness is about, you can use Tapping, along with gentle guidance, to help him/her to pinpoint the source of his/her sadness.

Child Tapping: What Am I Sad About?

If your child is unsure why s/he is sad, begin Tapping through the points with him/her as you ask a few questions, allowing time between each question for your child to share what comes to mind.

If s/he needs to cry, let him/her experience that release, and return to Tapping when s/he is ready.

You can ask questions like:

- When did you start feeling sad?
- Where were you when you began feeling sad?
- Were you alone or with someone when you started feeling sad?
- Did something happen (or not happen) that made you feel sad?
- Where do you feel your sadness in your body?

The answers to these questions are your Tapping targets. Tap with your child on releasing each one until his/her sadness is gone.

If Tapping through the points while asking questions like these doesn't produce an answer to explain what your child is sad about, you can also lead him/her through some rounds of Tapping on these questions. That Tapping might look something like this:

Karate Chop *(Repeat 3 times)*: Even though I'm not sure what I'm sad about, I'm a great kid and I'm okay.

Eyebrow: This sadness

Side of Eye: I'm not sure why I feel it

Under Eye: What am I sad about?

Under Nose: This sadness

Under Mouth: I don't know why I feel sad

Collarbone: What am I sad about?

Under Arm: This sadness

Top of Head: I can feel it in my body

Eyebrow: This sadness

Side of Eye: Where did it come from?

Under Eye: This sadness

Under Nose: Why do I feel it?

Under Mouth: This sadness

Collarbone: I'm not sure why I feel it

Under Arm: I wish I knew

Top of Head: It's okay that I don't know

Eyebrow: I do feel this sadness

Side of Eye: I feel it in my body

Under Eye: Why do I feel this sadness?

Under Nose: Maybe I can let myself see why

Under Mouth: Maybe I can let myself understand why I feel sad

Collarbone: It's safe to feel this sadness

Under Arm: And it's safe to let myself see why I'm feeling sad

Top of Head: It's safe to understand why I'm feeling this sadness

Take a deep breath, and see if your child wants to share any thoughts, ideas or memories that came to mind. If so, let him/her share. If not, keep Tapping until s/he gets more clarity.

Releasing Sadness

Once your child is aware of the reason for his/her sadness, you can then tap on releasing it.

If there's a specific event s/he is sad about, like being rejected, for instance, you may want to use the "Tell the Story" technique (see page 103) to release the event.

If your child is sad about a situation, like a friend moving away, for example, you can tap on his/her sadness around that situation.

Child Tapping: **Releasing Sadness about a Situation**

First ask your child to rate the intensity of his/her sadness, either on a scale of 0 to 10 or using the "this much" method of measurement.

Note: If at any point, your child needs to cry, let him/her experience that release, and return to Tapping when s/he is ready.

Take a deep breath, and begin by Tapping 3 times on the Karate Chop point.

Karate Chop *(Repeat 3 times)*: Even though I feel so much sadness about <reason for sadness>, I'm a great kid and I'm okay.

Eyebrow: This sadness

Side of Eye: I feel it in my heart

Under Eye: And I feel it in my body

Under Nose: So sad about <REASON>

Under Mouth: This sadness

Collarbone: It feels so big

Under Arm: It hurts

Top of Head: It's safe to let it out now

Eyebrow: It's safe to feel this sadness now

Side of Eye: I'm safe feeling this sadness

Under Eye: Even though it hurts

Under Nose: It's safe to let myself feel it now

Under Mouth: It hurts so badly

Collarbone: This sadness

Under Arm: It feels so big

Top of Head: It feels so heavy

Eyebrow: I can let myself feel it all now

Side of Eye: It's safe to feel this sadness now

Under Eye: And it's safe to let it go now

Under Nose: I'm safe feeling this sadness

Under Mouth: And I'm safe letting it go

Collarbone: I'm safe without this sadness

Under Arm: I don't have to push it away

Top of Head: I can just let it go now

Take a deep breath together and check back in with your child on the intensity of his/her sadness. Keep Tapping until s/he gets the desired relief.

Note: If your child's sadness is due to grief, trauma and/or other intense experiences, s/he may need to tap through those experiences. For more details on how to do that, refer to the appropriate section in this book, such as Grief, "Little t" Trauma or "Big T" Trauma. Extreme sadness may also be linked to multiple layers of experience, emotion and belief that need to be tapped through before the sadness can be fully released. Let the process unfold naturally, and continue talking and Tapping with your child as often as possible.

Child Tapping: **Feeling More Joy**

When your child has released most or all of his/her sadness, you can also do some positive rounds of Tapping on allowing your child to feel more joy.

Note: For general positive Tapping like this, it's okay to skip the rating step and go straight to Tapping. Also feel free to dance, skip and jump around while you tap!

Take a deep breath, and begin by Tapping 3 times on the Karate Chop point.

Karate Chop *(Repeat 3 times)*: Even though I sometimes feel sad or mad or scared, I can let myself feel joy and happiness, too!

Eyebrow: Sometimes I feel sad

Side of Eye: Sometimes I feel mad or scared

Under Eye: But I can feel joy!

Under Nose: I can feel happiness!

Under Mouth: And I can feel excitement!

Collarbone: So many fun things I can feel

Under Arm: It's safe to let myself feel it all

Top of Head: I'm a great kid!

Eyebrow: And I can let myself feel all of my feelings

Side of Eye: I can feel light

Under Eye: I can feel sunshine-y

Under Nose: I can feel rainbow-y

Under Mouth: And smiley, too!

Collarbone: It's fun to feel all these ways!

Under Arm: I'm a great kid

Top of Head: And I can let myself feel all these different ways

Eyebrow: I can feel like a fluffy, poufy cloud

Side of Eye: And like a goofy, cuckoo clown

Under Eye: I can dance

Under Nose: And I can jump

Under Mouth: I can feel happy

Collarbone: And I can feel super-duper excited!

Under Arm: I'm a great kid

Top of Head: And I'm safe feeling *all* of these different ways!

Keep Tapping if you like, or just go with the flow of whatever energy or mood your child now has.

TAPPING WITH YOUR CHILD: GRIEF

Grief is such an intense and personal journey that it's often hard to talk about. The kind of sadness we feel when we are grieving is incredibly powerful, and it may never vanish completely. But it can and often does shift and transform in ways that allow sadness and joy to co-exist in more balanced proportions.

In working with adults and children on their grief, the goal is never to erase the sadness that people feel. I honestly don't know if that's even possible. Using Tapping, however, we can help ourselves to move through the grieving process, and also to relieve everyday stress, which is hugely helpful when you're grieving.

Tapping is also a great tool for getting more restful sleep and releasing the emotional charge of painful memories and more of the challenging symptoms that often accompany the grieving process.

Before we look at how to use Tapping with your child on their grief, let's do some Tapping on the stress and worry you may feel as a result of your child's grief. The most powerful thing you can give to your child in this painful time is your presence, and to do that, you first need to take care of yourself.

Adult Tapping: Releasing Grief-Related Stress

When you think about your child's grief, what do you feel most urgently—anxiety? Worry? Helplessness or despair? Notice the most intense emotion, and rate it on a scale of 0 to 10.

Then take a deep breath and begin by Tapping 3 times on the Karate Chop point:

Karate Chop *(Repeat 3 times)*: Even though I feel so sad that my heart is heavy with my own grief and worry about my child's grief, I love myself and accept the way I feel.

Eyebrow: All this sadness

Side of Eye: This deep, heavy sadness

Under Eye: It hurts so deeply

Under Nose: I don't know how to help my child

Under Mouth: So worried about how to help her/him through this

Collarbone: So overwhelmed by my own sadness

Under Arm: I don't know how to help her/him through this

Top of Head: I didn't want her/him to have to feel this

Eyebrow: All this sadness

Side of Eye: All this worry

Under Eye: It's all too much

Under Nose: I don't know how to get through this myself

Under Mouth: I don't know how to help her/him get through this

Collarbone: So worried about him/her

Under Arm: Just too much

Top of Head: Letting myself feel this overwhelm now

Eyebrow: And this worry about her/him

Side of Eye: We can get through this one moment at a time

Under Eye: There's no fix for this

Under Nose: It's a process

Under Mouth: We can get through it one moment at a time

Collarbone: We can feel the sadness

Under Arm: And get through it one moment at a time

Top of Head: We'll move through this one moment at a time

Take a deep breath, and keep Tapping until you get the desired relief.

Now that you've gotten relief, let's look at how to use Tapping with your child on the grief s/he is feeling.

Note: As always, when Tapping with your child, tailor your words to your child's age and experience.

Grief over a Loved One

This story is a personal one, and among my most intense experiences around grief.

The tragic shooting at Sandy Hook Elementary School on December 14, 2012, in my hometown of Newtown, CT, traumatized our entire community. During the years that have passed since, The Tapping Solution Foundation took shape, and it has worked with countless people affected by this incredible tragedy.

One of those deeply affected by the massacre at Sandy Hook was JT Lewis, whose little brother, Jesse, tragically lost his life that day. While Tapping with his mother, Scarlett, Dr. Lori Leyden noticed that JT, who was 12 years old at the time, was struggling as well.

Since JT was hesitant about Tapping originally, Lori felt he may find meaning in talking with the PROJECT LIGHT ambassadors, who were victims of the genocide in Rwanda and had also lost family members to senseless violence. After years of doing healing work in Rwanda herself, Lori was in close contact with them.

A Skype call was arranged, and with the help of a translator JT spent more than 90 minutes talking to and Tapping with Chantal and Matthew, two of the Rwandans who had witnessed their relatives being murdered when they were children. Throughout their long call, JT remained engaged and willing to share his own experiences.

After a month of school absence, and nearly two months exhibiting very understandable signs of depression and anger, that evening JT began preparing to return to school. Since his Skype call with Mathew and Chantal, he had decided to give a presentation at school about how important it is to care about people around the world who have it worse than we do. In order to prepare, he spent that evening writing his speech.

In the months that followed, JT started a foundation, Newtown Helps Rwanda. As a result of the money raised, his foundation was able to send Betty, a Rwandan who had also survived the genocide, to university. In the years since, JT has also done some public appearances and radio interviews. His sadness may not be gone, but he has found a more constructive outlet for his grief.

We were fortunate to capture JT's Tapping experience on video, and he and his mother graciously agreed to let us share it in hopes of helping others traumatized by the loss of a loved one. To watch that movie, visit http://www.tappingsolutionfoundation.org/projectlight.

Child Tapping: Processing Grief over Losing a Loved One

To begin, have your child share how s/he is feeling. If it feels helpful, ask him/her to rate the intensity of his/her emotions, either on a 0 to 10 scale or the "this much" method of measurement. If the rating step feels disruptive, it's fine to skip it.

Take a deep breath together, and then begin by Tapping 3 times on the Karate Chop point:

Karate Chop *(Repeat 3 times)*: I have so much sadness in my heart, but I'm a great kid and I'm going to be okay.

Eyebrow: So much sadness

Side of Eye: So much heavy feeling in my heart

Under Eye: Nothing feels okay right now

Under Nose: So much sadness

Under Mouth: I feel it in my heart

Collarbone: I miss them so much

Under Arm: So much heavy feeling in my body

Top of Head: I miss them so much

Eyebrow: So much heavy sadness

Side of Eye: It's okay to feel it

Under Eye: I miss them so much

Under Nose: I feel so sad

Under Mouth: It feels so heavy

Collarbone: So sad

Under Arm: It's okay to feel this

Top of Head: I miss them so much

Eyebrow: So sad right now

Side of Eye: It's okay to feel this

Under Eye: We had so much fun together

Under Nose: And I'm a great kid

Under Mouth: Everything's going to be okay

Collarbone: Even though this heavy feeling doesn't feel okay

Under Arm: I'm a great kid

Top of Head: And everything's going to be okay

Keep Tapping until you sense that your child feels some relief.

Take a deep breath. Ask your child to rate his/her feelings again. Keep Tapping for as long as you like, or until your child gets the desired relief.

Connecting with Others, Receiving Support

In addition to relieving post-traumatic grief, Tapping can help trauma survivors to connect with others and seek out additional forms of healing. For JT, Tapping acted like a conduit, allowing him to share his experience with others who had suffered similarly, and then to take action on their behalf. Those connections and actions are healing unto themselves, and have given JT a sense of purpose that had been missing since his brother's death.

Child Tapping: Opening to Support and Community after Loss

In order to protect themselves, people often withdraw from others after experiencing a major loss. Unfortunately, the resulting isolation often can amplify grief and increase stress.

Let's look at how to use Tapping with your child to help him/her open up to receiving support and connection from people who can empathize with loss, which is itself a traumatic experience.

First, talk to your child about how isolated s/he is feeling and give that experience a number of intensity on a scale of 0 to 10.

Then take a deep breath. We'll begin by Tapping 3 times on the Karate Chop point.

> **Karate Chop** *(Repeat 3 times)*: Even though I feel so alone, I'm a great kid and I'm okay.

> **Eyebrow:** I feel so alone

> **Side of Eye:** So isolated by what happened

> **Under Eye:** No one understands

> **Under Nose:** I can't be around people

> **Under Mouth:** I can't talk about this

> **Collarbone:** I feel so alone

> **Under Arm:** So isolated by this trauma

> **Top of Head:** I have to protect myself

Eyebrow: I can't be with other people

Side of Eye: No one understands what this is like

Under Eye: I feel so alone

Under Nose: So isolated

Under Mouth: I can't talk about this

Collarbone: I can't face this

Under Arm: No one understands

Top of Head: I feel so alone

Eyebrow: Other people have been through this, too

Side of Eye: Maybe I can open up to the idea of connecting with them

Under Eye: Maybe I can seek out people who do understand

Under Nose: And feel less alone

Under Mouth: It's okay to feel scared about this

Collarbone: I can take it slowly

Under Arm: I can find people who get it

Top of Head: It's safe to receive support from others who understand

Take a deep breath now, and ask your child how intense his/her feeling of being alone is now. Give it a number, and keep Tapping until s/he gets the desired relief.

Losing a Grandparent

Coming to grips with the loss of a grandparent is a common, and often heart-breaking, experience for children. While the initial passing can be difficult, the grieving process often also extends into other times, such as weekends or holidays when your child may be used to visiting or talking to grandpa or grandma.

Child Tapping: Processing Grief over Losing a Grandparent

Each person's journey through grief is different. The goal with Tapping on grief is to allow your child to feel and express his/her emotions, rather than releasing them. This naturally takes time, but by using Tapping to allow challenging emotions to arise, your child will be better able to move through the grieving process.

With grief, it's normal to need to tap repeatedly with your child when sadness and other related emotions arise. As always, don't hesitate to pause your Tapping if your child needs to cry, cuddle or hug.

To begin, ask your child, how s/he is feeling. If it doesn't feel disruptive, rate the intensity of his/her primary emotion, either on a scale of 0 to 10 or using the "this much" method of measurement.

Karate Chop *(Repeat 3 times)*: Even though I'm so sad that grandma/grandpa has passed on, I'm a great kid and I'm okay.

Eyebrow: I miss him/her so much

Side of Eye: I don't understand how s/he could be gone

Under Eye: I'm so sad

Under Nose: How is this possible?

Under Mouth: All this sadness

Collarbone: I feel it in my heart

Under Arm: I feel it in my body

Top of Head: It hurts so much

Eyebrow: I want grandma/grandpa back!

Side of Eye: I'm so, so sad

Under Eye: I miss him/her so much

Under Nose: This doesn't feel possible

Under Mouth: I want to be with her/him

Collarbone: I'm so, so sad

Under Arm: I can't believe this is happening

Top of Head: All this sadness

Eyebrow: It's doesn't feel okay to feel this

Side of Eye: It feels like too much sadness

Under Eye: But it's safe to feel this sadness

Under Nose: Even though it feels so intense

Under Mouth: All this sadness

Collarbone: I feel it everywhere

Under Arm: It's safe to feel this sadness now

Top of Head: It's safe to let myself feel this sadness

Check back in with your child on how s/he is feeling now. Since the grieving process is so particular to each person and circumstance, let your child set the pace of your Tapping. Keep Tapping for as long as your child desires.

Losing a Pet

Riggsy had cancer. The elder of the two dogs in my brother Alex's family, Riggsy's pain seemed to be getting much worse. The tumors in his mouth had also grown large, and he could no longer navigate stairs or play and run as he always had. Wanting to give him peace, my brother and his wife, Karen, made the difficult decision to put Riggsy to sleep.

A deeply intuitive dog, Riggsy had always been an important part of the family. When you'd had a bad day, Riggsy always appeared by your side, ready to comfort and reassure you. For their son Malakai, who is now 8 years old, Riggsy had also been a first best friend.

Once the decision had been made to put Riggsy down, Alex and Karen began looking into how to best share the news with Malakai, as well as with their other son Lucas, who was 3 years old at the time. They were advised not to tell the boys that Riggsy was going to sleep, since that tends to confuse kids. Instead, they explained the process in simple terms, saying he would seem to be going to sleep, but that really Riggsy was going to die. They then reassured the boys that Riggsy would be comfortable and happy, and that it wouldn't hurt him.

Wanting to involve Malakai and Lucas in the process, each family member then made a heart-shaped card. They talked about their happiest memo-ies of Riggsy play-fighting with their other dog, Leo, fetching sticks, going on walks and more. Karen and Alex helped the boys write those memories on their cards, which they planned to bury with Riggsy's body. Wanting to keep a copy of his card, Malakai then made a duplicate card that he hung on the wall in his bedroom.

They gathered together in the backyard to bury Riggsy's body. Each person had a white rose, which they placed by Riggsy's body, along with their card. They all helped to cover his body.

On that day and during the weeks and months that followed, the family continued to talk about Riggsy. Both Alex and Karen made a point of allowing the boys to feel and express their sadness, and to tap, when they wanted to, on it being okay to feel that sadness.

One day about six months after Riggsy was put to sleep, Malakai shared how much he still missed Riggsy, and how difficult his absence still was. Rather than trying to fix or release his sadness, Karen and Alex once again let him speak about his feelings. Without trying to reassure Malakai that Riggsy was happy now, and without ever asking him to let go of his emotions or move on, they simply created a safe space so that Malakai could feel his sadness when it overcame him. Now they often still tell stories about Riggsy, and although time hasn't removed the sadness entirely, it has lessened its intensity.

Child Tapping: Processing Grief over Losing a Pet

Once again, the goal here is to support your child in moving through the grieving process.

The following Tapping script focuses on sadness, but as always, tap on your child's present-moment experience, whether it's actual grief, or related symptoms, which could be physical pain, sleep issues, anger or other. Since children are often more aware of the physical sensations, also ask them what they're feeling in their body.

To begin, have your child tell you how they're feeling, and then rate it either on a 0 to 10 scale or using the "this much" method of measurement.

Take a deep breath together, and then begin by Tapping 3 times on the Karate Chop point:

Karate Chop *(Repeat 3 times)*: I have so much sadness in my heart, but I'm a great kid and I'm going to be okay.

Eyebrow: So much sadness

Side of Eye: So much heavy feeling in my heart

Under Eye: Nothing feels okay right now

Under Nose: So much sadness about missing <pet name>

Under Mouth: I feel it in my heart

Collarbone: My tummy doesn't feel good

Under Arm: So much heavy feeling in my body

Top of Head: I want <pet name> back

Eyebrow: So much heavy sadness

Side of Eye: It's okay to feel it

Under Eye: We had so much fun together

Under Nose: And I miss <pet name> so much

Under Mouth: It makes me so sad

Collarbone: It feels so heavy

Under Arm: It's okay to feel this

Top of Head: We had so much fun together

Eyebrow: And I'm so sad about missing <pet name>

Side of Eye: It's okay to feel this

Under Eye: We had so much fun together

Under Nose: And I'm a great kid

Under Mouth: Everything's going to be okay

Collarbone: Even though this heavy feeling doesn't feel okay

Under Arm: I'm a great kid

Top of Head: And everything's going to be okay

Take a deep breath. When your child is ready, have him/her rate his/her feelings again. If s/he is willing, keep Tapping until s/he gets the desired relief.

TAPPING WITH YOUR CHILD: DEPRESSION

Children are often moody, cycling easily in and out of "the blues." But what happens when feeling "the blues," or even constant moodiness, becomes the norm for your child?

Depression manifests in children in different ways, but often includes a significant change, or several changes, in behavior. For instance, your once out-going child might suddenly have no interest in playing with friends, or your physically active child may start sleeping all the time or become lethargic and irritable.

Once depression takes hold, it can quickly shift into a downward cycle that is hard to disrupt. As one example, let's say your child starts feeling depressed and begins sleeping more. As a result she spends less time with friends, who feel rejected by her, and eventually stop inviting her along. That, in turn, makes your child feel unloved, which then adds to her depression—and just like that, the cycle self-perpetuates.

To make matters worse, just when your child most needs your love and support, s/he feels too depressed to voice his/her needs and desires.

Tapping is a great way to help your child get his/her emotions and energy moving again. Before we look at how to use Tapping with a depressed child, however, we'll begin with Tapping on the stress and worry you may feel as a result of your child's depression.

IS MY CHILD DEPRESSED?

Recognizing depression in children isn't always easy. While there are different kinds of depression, and a long list of relevant symptoms, depression is generally defined as more than being "down in the dumps."

Sadness is often mistaken for depression, but sadness is a healthy, although unpleasant, emotional response to experiences. While sadness can lead to depressive behavior and may even last for longer periods of time, it's a definitive emotional response to something or someone.

Unlike sadness, depression is often characterized by emotional numbness, as well as apathy, low energy and chronic moodiness.

Teenagers in particular commonly experience periods where they withdraw and may not seem like their "normal" selves. While these changes in mood and behavior can turn into long-term depression, they can also be phases that pass or smooth out naturally within a period of days or perhaps a couple of weeks.

Unlike grief, PTSD and other challenging but normal responses to events and circumstances, depression often seems like an ongoing case of "the blues" that doesn't have a clear cause.

While depression has been linked to the brain, it's important also to remember that the brain is neuroplastic, meaning that it's capable of transforming. Tapping, as well as physical exercise, wholesome nutrition, improved sleep and other positive habits support positive changes in the brain and body.

Adult Tapping: Releasing Stress around Your Child's Depression

Watching your child suffer with depression is painful and frustrating for parents, who want nothing more than to resolve their child's pain and hopelessness. Before you try Tapping with your child on his/her depression, it's important to tap on your own emotions first.

To start, notice which emotion(s) you feel most intensely when you think about your child's depression—fear, anxiety, anger, shame? Focus on your primary emotion and give it a number of intensity on a scale of 0 to 10.

I'll focus on fear and anxiety, but as always, focus your Tapping on your experience.

Take a deep breath, and begin by Tapping 3 times on the Karate Chop point.

Karate Chop *(Repeat 3 times)*: Even though I'm so scared and anxious about my child's depression, I deeply and completely love and accept myself.

Eyebrow: S/he is so depressed

Side of Eye: It's so painful to watch

Under Eye: I'm so afraid for him/her

Under Nose: So anxious about his/her depression

Under Mouth: I need to fix this

Collarbone: But I'm not sure how

Under Arm: I don't know if s/he will let me help

Top of Head: I'm so scared

Eyebrow: So anxious

Side of Eye: I feel so hopeless

Under Eye: I need to be able to fix this

Under Nose: I need to do something to help

Under Mouth: All this fear

Collarbone: All this anxiety

Under Arm: His/her depression

Top of Head: It's overwhelming

Eyebrow: It's okay to feel this way

Side of Eye: I can trust this process

Under Eye: I can relax even though things don't seem okay right now

Under Nose: I can trust this process

Under Mouth: It's safe to feel safe

Collarbone: It's safe to relax now

Under Arm: Letting go of this fear and anxiety now

Top of Head: Feeling relaxed and at peace now

Take a deep breath. How intense is your primary emotion now? Keep Tapping until you get the desired relief.

IS MY CHILD'S DEPRESSION MY FAULT?

Many loving, caring parents wonder if they're to blame for their child's depression. The answer is no. Depression isn't something you wanted for your child, and not something for which you should blame yourself.

Since awareness is critical to the treatment process, it is important to know that, according to the Anxiety and Depression Association of America[2], children of depressed parents are at higher risk for depression themselves. That doesn't mean that you're at fault, however. Instead, it's a reason to notice any depressive tendencies, as well as persistent changes in mood and/or behavior, in yourself as well as your child.

Depression can be challenging, but it is treatable. Recognizing that your child may be suffering from depression is a huge step forward. If you yourself have suffered or currently are suffering from depression, be sure to use Tapping on your own, as well.

Now that you've had an experience, let's look at some of the ways that you can use Tapping to support your child in overcoming his/her depression.

Note: As always, when Tapping with your child, tailor your words to your child's age and experience.

Child/Teenager Tapping: Shedding "The Blues"

If your child is suffering from "the blues," s/he may seem disengaged, no longer interested in the people, places and activities that once energized her/him. Tapping can help to reignite your child's spark, and also to give him/her insight into the deeper emotions that may be (dis)coloring his/her inner and outer worlds.

If your child is willing, have him/her rate how "blue" or "blah" s/he is feeling, either on a 0 to 10 scale or using the "this much" method of measurement.

Take a deep breath and begin by Tapping 3 times on the Karate Chop point.

Karate Chop *(Repeat 3 times):* Even though nothing feels good anymore, I love myself and accept how I feel.

Eyebrow: This darkness

Side of Eye: Nothing feels good anymore

Under Eye: Things are so bleak

Under Nose: Nothing feels worthwhile anymore

Under Mouth: All this darkness

Collarbone: It's too much

Under Arm: This darkness

Top of Head: I can't escape it

Eyebrow: This darkness

Side of Eye: I can't shed it

Under Eye: It's overwhelming

Under Nose: This darkness

Under Mouth: I feel it everywhere

Collarbone: It won't go away

Under Arm: What's this darkness really about?

Top of Head: Why won't this darkness go away?

Eyebrow: It's safe to feel this darkness

Side of Eye: And it's safe to let it fade away

Under Eye: I can see what's beneath it

Under Nose: It's safe to feel what's there

Under Mouth: It's safe to see and feel it all

Collarbone: It feels big

Under Arm: But it's not bigger than I am

Top of Head: It's safe to let this darkness fade away now

Take a deep breath together. Check back in with your child on how intense the "blah" feels now. Keep Tapping until s/he gets the desired relief.

Child/Teenager Tapping: Moving beyond Irritability

If your child's depression is making him/her irritable, Tapping is a great way to calm that urge.

First, if your child is willing, ask him/her to rate how irritable that s/he feels, either on a 0 to 10 scale or using the "this much" method of measurement.

Take a deep breath, and begin by Tapping 3 times on the Karate Chop point.

Karate Chop *(Repeat 3 times)*: Even though I feel so irritable, I can't be around anyone or anything, I deeply and completely love and accept myself.

Eyebrow: I feel so irritable

Side of Eye: People irritate me

Under Eye: Things irritate me

Under Nose: So irritable right now

Under Mouth: It's maddening!

Collarbone: It's all so annoying

Under Arm: I can't stand it

Top of Head: It needs to stop

Eyebrow: It all needs to go away

Side of Eye: I need to be left alone

Under Eye: So irritable right now

Under Nose: It's overwhelming feeling this irritable

Under Mouth: Nothing feels fun

Collarbone: Can't be around anyone or anything

Under Arm: All this irritability

Top of Head: It's hard to live with

Eyebrow: Maybe I don't have to

Side of Eye: Maybe I can let myself feel it all now

Under Eye: And then let it all go

Under Nose: It's safe to let this irritability go now

Under Mouth: I'm not enjoying it

Collarbone: I don't need it

Under Arm: It's safe to let it go now

Top of Head: It's safe to relax and feel calmer now

Take a deep breath together. Check back in with your child on how irritable s/he is feeling. Keep Tapping until s/he gets the desired relief.

Child/Teenager Tapping: Moving beyond Hopelessness

Feeling hopeless is one of the most heartbreaking parts of depression since that sense of hopelessness can strip away the potential for joy, love, connection and fun.

Let's do some Tapping now on stepping out of that darkness and regaining hope.

If your child is willing, ask him/her to rate his/her sense of hopelessness, either on a scale of 0 to 10 or using the "this much" method of measurement.

Take a deep breath, and begin by Tapping 3 times on the Karate Chop point.

Karate Chop *(Repeat 3 times)*: Even though I feel so hopeless, like nothing's ever going to get better, I'm okay.

Eyebrow: This hopelessness

Side of Eye: It feels so definite

Under Eye: Like I can't change or move it

Under Nose: This hopelessness

Under Mouth: It's so heavy

Collarbone: Nothing feels worth it

Under Arm: I can't shake it

Top of Head: It feels so real and so dark

Eyebrow: This hopelessness

Side of Eye: I can't shake it

Under Eye: It's so thick and so dark

Under Nose: What's it all about?

Under Mouth: This hopelessness

Collarbone: When did it start?

Under Arm: Why can't I shake it?

Top of Head: This hopelessness

Eyebrow: Maybe it's not permanent

Side of Eye: Maybe I don't have to believe it's real

Under Eye: Maybe I can shake it off

Under Nose: Maybe I can let go of this hopelessness now

Under Mouth: It's safe to let go of this hopelessness

Collarbone: It's not making me happy

Under Arm: It's safe to let it go now

Top of Head: It's safe to relax and feel hopeful now

Take a deep breath together. Check back in with your child on his/her hopelessness now. Keep Tapping until s/he gets the desired relief.

Child/Teenager Tapping: "All I Want to Do Is _____"

One symptom of depression is spending most waking hours doing one or two things, such as watching television, sleeping, eating or playing video games.

If your child has fallen into a similarly unhealthy pattern, Tapping can help him/her to move beyond it.

First ask your child to rate how resistant s/he feels about doing an activity s/he used to enjoy, whether it's riding a bike, playing with a friend, creating art/music or other.

I'll focus on watching television, but as always, tailor your Tapping to your child's experience.

Take a deep breath, and begin by Tapping 3 times on the Karate Chop point.

Karate Chop (*Repeat 3 times*): Even though I don't want to do anything else—I only want to watch TV—I'm okay.

Eyebrow: I don't want to do anything else

Side of Eye: Watching TV is the only thing I want to do

Under Eye: Nothing else feels comforting

Under Nose: I don't want to go outside

Under Mouth: I don't want to play

Collarbone: I don't want to see friends

Under Arm: I only want to watch TV

Top of Head: I don't want to do anything else

Eyebrow: Nothing else sounds fun

Side of Eye: Everything else sounds hard

Under Eye: I only want to watch TV

Under Nose: I'm watching a lot of TV

Under Mouth: It's all I want to do

Collarbone: That's okay

Under Arm: It's a lot of TV

Top of Head: Maybe I could go outside for a few minutes

Eyebrow: Or talk to someone

Side of Eye: I can take a break from TV

Under Eye: And come back later

Under Nose: I can do something that's not TV

Under Mouth: I can try it for a little bit

Collarbone: It's safe to do something else

Under Arm: It's safe to talk and be with people

Top of Head: Letting go of this need to watch TV all the time

Take a deep breath together. Check back in with your child on how resistant s/he feels about doing something different, such as going outside, helping you with a project or interacting with friends or neighbors. Keep Tapping until s/he gets the desired relief.

Depression can be a complex condition, and recovery is often an ongoing process. As often as s/he is willing, tap with your child on his/her emotions, experience and behavior. As always, if your child's depression persists or worsens, seek out professional support.

TAPPING WITH YOUR CHILD: GUILT

Guilt is an interesting emotion. Unlike shame, which tarnishes the sense of self (*"I am* a bad person"*) guilt points to mistakes or missteps a person made (*"I did/said* a bad thing, and now I feel badly about it."*) Although guilt can be difficult to experience, it's generally viewed as a healthy emotional response to errors in judgment, action or inaction.

When guilt is used as a reason to accept responsibility and take appropriate action, such as apologizing for hurting someone's feelings, guilt can positively impact self-esteem and relationships. Some studies[3] have even demonstrated a link between being prone to guilt and leadership skills, in part because guilt encourages people to take responsibility for and resolve mistakes that they've made.

Guilt only becomes a liability when it's held onto for too long, past the point where it is constructive. In this section, we'll look at some different kinds of guilt, and how you can help your child to release it with Tapping. As always, the best place to start is by Tapping on your own stress and emotions, which is what we'll do next.

Adult Tapping: **Releasing Parental Guilt**

At one point or another, we all experience some kind of guilt around parenting. Whether it's because of absences, or mistakes we believe we've made, we all feel some level of parental guilt.

To begin, focus on any parenting guilt you feel currently or have felt recently. Rate the intensity of that guilt on a scale of 0 to 10.

Take a deep breath and begin by Tapping 3 times on the Karate Chop point.

Karate Chop *(Repeat 3 times)*: Even though I feel all this guilt, I deeply and completely love and accept myself.

Eyebrow: All this guilt

Side of Eye: It feels like my fault

Under Eye: This guilt

Under Nose: It's overwhelming

Under Mouth: It feels so heavy

Collarbone: This guilt

Under Arm: I feel like this is my fault

Top of Head: So much guilt

Eyebrow: It's overwhelming

Side of Eye: It feels like my fault

Under Eye: All this guilt

Under Nose: I meant to do better

Under Mouth: My child deserves better

Collarbone: This guilt

Under Arm: It's a heavy load

Top of Head: Maybe I can put it down now

Eyebrow: I can take full responsibility for my mistake

Side of Eye: And apologize or do what I need to do to make things right

Under Eye: It's safe to let go of this guilt now

Under Nose: It's safe to let myself move on

Under Mouth: My mistakes don't define me

Collarbone: And I don't need this guilt to avoid this mistake in the future

Under Arm: It's safe to let go of this guilt now

Top of Head: Letting myself feel safe and guilt-free now

Take a deep breath. Rate the intensity of your parenting guilt now. Keep Tapping until you get the desired relief.

Now that you've had an experience, let's look at how you can help your child to use Tapping to release guilt s/he may be feeling.

Note: As always, when Tapping with your child, tailor your words to your child's age and experience.

Child Tapping: "I Lied/I Did a Bad Thing"

If your child is feeling guilty about making a bad choice, whether by lying, saying or doing something hurtful or for any other reason, first let him/her talk about and express how s/he is feeling without judgment or comment.

Note: As always, if your child's actions cause an emotional response in you, tap on releasing that response first, before Tapping with your child.

Next ask him/her to rate the intensity of the guilt s/he is feeling, either on a scale of 0 to 10 or using the "this much" method of measurement.

As always, tailor your Tapping to your child's experience and words.

Take a deep breath and begin by Tapping 3 times on the Karate Chop point.

Karate Chop *(Repeat 3 times)*: Even though I feel so much guilt about what I did, I'm a great kid and I'm okay.

Eyebrow: This guilt

Side of Eye: I feel really badly

Under Eye: I made a bad choice

Under Nose: I feel really guilty about it

Under Mouth: This guilt

Collarbone: I made a bad choice

Under Arm: I feel really badly about it

Top of Head: This guilt

Eyebrow: It feels so heavy

Side of Eye: I made a mistake

Under Eye: What I did/said was wrong

Under Nose: I feel really badly about it

Under Mouth: Maybe I can fix it

Collarbone: I can do the right thing

Under Arm: And I can let go of this guilt

Top of Head: This guilt feels so heavy

Eyebrow: I can let it go now

Side of Eye: I made a mistake, but now I can make a good choice

Under Eye: And I can let go of this guilt

Under Nose: I made a mistake

Under Mouth: But I'm not a bad person

Collarbone: I can make a good choice now

Under Arm: And I can let go of this guilt

Top of Head: It's safe to relax and let go of this guilt now

Take a deep breath together, and check back in with your child on the intensity of his/her guilt now. Keep Tapping until s/he gets the desired relief.

When your child is ready, you can also offer to tap through the points while brainstorming together about good choices s/he can make now and in the future. You can also help your child to come up with his/her own solutions by asking open-ended questions like:

- What amends do you need/want to make?

- How and when will you make those amends?

- How might you handle this situation next time, if it arises again?

Child Tapping: "I Didn't Do Enough"

Sometimes we feel guilty about an action we didn't take or an effort we didn't make, especially when our lack of response negatively impacts others.

For instance, if your child feels guilty about not playing hard enough in a championship game his/her team lost, or for not speaking up to defend a friend, s/he can use Tapping to release that guilt and assume a healthy amount of responsibility for his/her inaction.

To begin, ask your child to rate the intensity of his/her guilt, either on a 0 to 10 scale or using the "this much" method of measurement.

Take a deep breath and begin by Tapping 3 times on the Karate Chop point.

Karate Chop *(Repeat 3 times)*: Even though I feel so guilty about not doing/saying enough, I love myself and accept how I feel.

Eyebrow: This guilt

Side of Eye: I should have tried harder/done more

Under Eye: I feel really badly

Under Nose: I didn't do enough

Under Mouth: My inaction hurt people

Collarbone: And I feel really guilty about that

Under Arm: I didn't mean for anyone to get hurt

Top of Head: All this guilt

Eyebrow: I didn't mean for this to happen

Side of Eye: I feel really badly

Under Eye: My lack of effort/inaction hurt people

Under Nose: And I feel like it's all my fault

Under Mouth: I didn't mean for things to turn out this way

Collarbone: Maybe I made a bad choice

Under Arm: But I'm still great

Top of Head: I don't have to be perfect to be great

Eyebrow: I'm great!

Side of Eye: And I can let go of this guilt now

Under Eye: I don't have to be perfect to be great

Under Nose: It's safe to let this go now

Under Mouth: Releasing this guilt now

Collarbone: I'm great!

Under Arm: And I don't have to be perfect

Top of Head: I can relax and feel good now

Take a deep breath together and check back in with your child on the intensity of his/her guilt now. Keep Tapping until s/he gets the desired relief.

Again, if your child is willing, it's a great idea to ask open-ended questions that prompt him/her to come up with solutions. For instance, you might ask questions like:

- Why do you think you didn't *action*/try harder/help out?
  - If your child expresses another emotion, such as fear of failing or speaking up, be sure to tap on releasing that.

- What can you do to make amends?

- How and when will you make those amends?

- If a similar situation happens again, what could you do differently next time?

Child Tapping: "I Shouldn't Be This Good at School/Sports/Etc."

If your child is suffering from guilt due to his/her performance being better than others', first know that his/her guilt is considered to be a less traumatic form of survivor's guilt.

This type of survivor's guilt is relatively common, and has been documented in people who experience a high level of success in one or several areas. As one example, first-generation college students have been shown to suffer from guilt that their parents and perhaps their sibling(s) couldn't or can't attend college. Some find their guilt so intolerable that they resort to unconscious self-sabotage, often in the form of behavior that ensures their own failure.

To begin Tapping on releasing this guilt, first ask your child to rate the intensity of his/her guilt around performing better than others, either on a scale of 0 to 10 or using the "this much" method of measurement.

Take a deep breath and begin by Tapping 3 times on the Karate Chop point.

Karate Chop *(Repeat 3 times)*: Even though I feel all this guilt about doing well, I love myself and accept how I feel.

Eyebrow: All this guilt

Side of Eye: I feel badly

Under Eye: I'm not trying to make anyone look bad

Under Nose: I work hard, though!

Under Mouth: I hate that I have to feel guilty about doing my best

Collarbone: Everyone else works hard, too

Under Arm: I'm not sure if I deserve to do this well

Top of Head: This guilt

Eyebrow: It feels so heavy

Side of Eye: It's not my fault that I do well

Under Eye: I can't control how others perform

Under Nose: I'm just doing my best

Under Mouth: That's a good thing!

Collarbone: I want to do my best

Under Arm: It feels good!

Top of Head: I'm not responsible for how other people do

Eyebrow: It's safe to let go of this guilt

Side of Eye: I can't control how others do

Under Eye: Releasing this guilt now

Under Nose: It's good to do my best!

Under Mouth: It's safe for me to feel worthy of my success

Collarbone: It's safe to appreciate my own success

Under Arm: It's safe for me to work hard and do well

Top of Head: It's safe to feel good about doing my best!

Take a deep breath together, and check back in with your child on the intensity of his/her guilt. Keep Tapping until s/he gets the desired relief.

RELEASING TRAUMATIC SURVIVOR'S GUILT

Traumatic survivor's guilt has been repeatedly documented in trauma survivors, including war veterans. This type of survivor's guilt is intensely traumatic, and can more easily morph into shame. It's also often tied to traumatic memories, emotions and beliefs.

If you or your child is navigating traumatic survivor's guilt, it's important to embark on a larger journey that addresses all facets of the trauma you and/or your child survived. Tapping can treat PTSD, survivor's guilt and other trauma symptoms more thoroughly and quickly than other treatments.

In cases of traumatic survivor's guilt, I highly recommend seeking support from a professional who can support you and/or your child through a trauma healing and recovery process. For a list of certified EFT professionals, visit http://thetappingsolution.com/eft-practitioners/.

TAPPING WITH YOUR CHILD: SHAME AND SELF-HATRED

"Shame is a soul-eating emotion."—Carl Jung

Burning shame. It's an accurate description of one of our most scarring emotions. A deep, often buried emotion, shame erodes our sense of self, creating beliefs like, "I am unworthy," "I am unlovable," "I am a failure/not good enough" and more.

Before we look more closely at shame, let's look further at how it differs from guilt. While guilt can be intense, it relates to something a person said or did, rather than who s/he is. As a result, even overwhelming guilt (*"I did* a bad thing") is often easier to heal than shame (*"I am* a bad person"). If guilt is left unhealed, of course, it can morph into shame.

Shame thrives in darkness, and it is incredibly painful to acknowledge and talk about. Even the act of feeling shame is thought to amplify shame. Not surprisingly, our natural response to shame is to avoid and hide it, which then allows it to intensify. How frustrating!

While shame can stem from trauma, such as abuse in childhood, there are other, subtler causes for it. As a culture, it's only relatively recently that we've become aware of what causes shame, and how it impacts self-image and child development. While statements like "you are a bad boy/girl" were commonplace among parents only a generation or two ago, we now understand that statements like that cause children to feel shame. Instead of using defining statements—"you are bad"—parenting experts recommend focusing on actions—"that was a bad choice"—in order to avoid creating shame.

As I've said, I'm not a parenting expert, but I do think it's important to ac-knowledge how new our understanding of shame is. Many of us heard shame-creating statements as children and may have unintentionally repeated them as parents. Our children may also feel shame as a result of social situations that we are unaware of. Whatever the causes, it's important to remember that shame *can* be healed. Tapping is a powerful way to shed light on shame, and that alone is healing.

As always, the best place to start is by Tapping on your own emotions, so before we look at how to tap with your child on releasing it, let's first tap on how you feel about your child's shame.

Adult Tapping: Releasing Angst over Your Child's Shame

Watching your child suffer from shame is painful for any parent, so before you tap with your child, it's important first to release any emotions *you* may feel around your child's shame.

First notice what primary emotion(s) you feel when you think about your child's shame. Give the emotion(s) a number of intensity on a scale of 0 to 10.

As always, tailor your Tapping to your own experience.

Take a deep breath, and begin by Tapping 3 times on the Karate Chop point.

Karate Chop *(Repeat 3 times)*: Even though I'm so scared this is all my fault, I've made so many mistakes, I deeply and completely love and accept myself.

Eyebrow: So worried about my child

Side of Eye: This shame s/he is feeling

Under Eye: What if it's all my fault?

Under Nose: I've made so many mistakes

Under Mouth: I'm so worried

Collarbone: And so scared

Under Arm: What if this is all my fault?

Top of Head: All this worry

Eyebrow: All this fear

Side of Eye: It breaks my heart that s/he feels this shame

Under Eye: I want him/her to see what I see

Under Nose: The amazing, wonderful child I see

Under Mouth: Why can't s/he see that?

Collarbone: This hurts so much

Under Arm: It hurts seeing him/her hurting so deeply

Top of Head: So scared and worried

Eyebrow: It's safe to feel all of this

Side of Eye: It's safe to feel all this worry and fear now

Under Eye: And it's safe to let it all go

Under Nose: We can heal together

Under Mouth: I can let this all go now

Collarbone: We can heal together

Under Arm: It's safe to feel hopeful now

Top of Head: It's safe to trust that we'll heal together

Take a deep breath and rate the intensity of your primary emotion(s) again now. Keep Tapping until you get the desired relief.

Now that you've had an experience, let's look at how to use Tapping to heal your child's shame.

Note: As always, when Tapping with your child, tailor your words to your child's age and experience.

"You're a Show-off!"

Name-calling is one way that kids can take on shame. For 12-year-old Kari, it happened one day at school when her teacher called her a show-off as she was organizing classmates to present a speech to a visiting teacher.

Arriving home from school that afternoon, Kari was in a foul, brooding mood. She explained that she felt overwhelmed by her teacher's accusation, and didn't know how to take it.

Recognizing the teacher's comment as shame-creating, Kari's mom immediately began to worry that feedback like this would dim her daughter's light and, over time, cause Kari to squash her innate leadership skills.

After calmly asking Kari if she wanted to do some Tapping on how she was feeling about her teacher's comment, they began to tap on what her teacher had said that day.

Before they'd even finished a single round of Tapping, Kari blurted out, "I'm glad my teacher called me a show-off!" Her mom asked her why and she explained that someday her teacher would see her on television and remember that she'd known Kari. "She'll be an old lady and she'll see me on her TV and say, 'That girl was a show-off in 6th grade, and now look at her, she's changing the world!'"

Confident that Kari had not internalized any shame as a result of her teacher's comment, her mom led her through a round of positive Tapping, and ended with a great big hug. By the end Kari was calm and happy, grateful for her experience at school that day and for Tapping with her mom.

Can you imagine a world in which all girls could feel this kind of confidence? Amazing! I love that Kari's mom jumped on the opportunity to prevent shame from taking root, and that Kari intuitively understood her own power to deflect, rather than internalize, her teacher's comment. By Tapping on the event, Kari anchored herself in her own power, rather than in self-doubt.

Child Tapping: Letting Go of "You're So _____" Remarks

If your child is experiencing shame due to a comment like "you're bossy," "you're a bad kid" or something similar, first ask him/her to focus on what was said and rate how true it feels, either on a scale of 0 to 10 or using the "this much" method of measurement.

Note: Kids often react to and interpret remarks differently than adults. If you're aware of negative remarks made to your child but aren't sure how s/he is feeling about it, ask him/her first how s/he feels about it. If s/he doesn't feel any shame or seem to be bothered by it, trust that there's no need to tap on it right now. If down the road shame becomes an issue, you can gently bring up the remark(s) again. As always, though, don't force your child to tap on anything unless s/he is willing.

When Tapping on a remark, it's important to repeat the comment numerous times while Tapping through the points. While I'll use "you're so bossy" below, tailor your own Tapping to the remark that was made to your child.

Take a deep breath and begin by Tapping 3 times on the Karate Chop point.

Karate Chop *(Repeat 3 times)*: Even though she said I'm so bossy, I'm a great kid and I'm okay.

Eyebrow: "You're so bossy"

Side of Eye: "You're so bossy"

Under Eye: That's what she said to me

Under Nose: "You're so bossy"

Under Mouth: It hurt my feelings

Collarbone: It made me feel sad

Under Arm: And now I feel mad about it, too!

Top of Head: That's not a nice thing to say

Eyebrow: I'm not bossy!

Side of Eye: I'm so mad about this

Under Eye: And so sad

Under Nose: It made me want to go away

Under Mouth: I didn't like it when she said that

Collarbone: I'm mad about it

Under Arm: And sad, too

Top of Head: I'm not bossy

Eyebrow: I have a lot of ideas

Side of Eye: I was sharing them

Under Eye: It's safe to share my ideas

Under Nose: Maybe I can do it more gently next time

Under Mouth: But that doesn't mean I'm bossy

Collarbone: I'm a great kid!

Under Arm: And I'm okay

Top of Head: I have lots of ideas and I love that about myself

Take a deep breath together, and check back in with your child on how true the remark feels now. Keep Tapping until s/he gets the desired relief.

Self-Esteem

How your child feels about him or herself is a reflection of his/her self-esteem, which is essentially your child's sense of self-worth.

Although the terms self-confidence and self-esteem are sometimes used interchangeably, they are not the same. Self-confidence relates to specific abilities, whereas self-esteem refers to how a person feels about him or herself. For example, a child may feel confident in her soccer abilities, but suffer from low self-esteem because of a fundamental belief that she is not good/pretty/lovable/smart enough. Similarly, a child may experience positive self-esteem, believing that he is loved and worthy, but suffer from low confidence in math.

Although they're different, self-esteem and self-confidence can feed on each other in positive, as well as negative, ways. For instance, a child's high self-confidence in soccer may boost her overall self-esteem. Conversely, long-lasting low confidence in math may eventually put a dent in self-esteem.

Depending on your child's current and past experiences, his/her self-esteem (and self-confidence!) will likely ebb and flow over time. While it's important to notice and respond to changes in a child's self-esteem, remember that some fluctuation is normal, and typically not a reason to panic. Needless to say, if you notice dramatic and/or long-lasting dips in your child's self-esteem, trust your instincts, and seek professional help if necessary.

If your child is suffering from decreased self-esteem, the most important thing you can give him or her is your open and loving presence. Watching your child in emotional pain, or hearing him/her say things like, "I'm dumb," "I'm not a good kid," or "I can't do anything right" is heartbreaking for any parent.

When your child says or does something that reflects his/her self-esteem challenges, what do you experience in your body? What emotions come up? Do you worry that your child has inherited your own self-esteem issues? How do you feel about yourself as a parent in those moments?

Your goal should never be to blame or shame yourself. Your goal is simply to be honest about how you're feeling, since that's the only way to transform it. If, for instance, your child's self-esteem challenges seem similar to self-esteem challenges that you yourself are facing or have faced in the past, recognize that there may be a connection. While your child's self-esteem challenges are not your fault, know that by using Tapping yourself, you can gradually address your own self-worth issues, and in so doing, help your child to heal over time.

Child Tapping: **Releasing Stress from Self-Esteem Challenges**

If your child is struggling with self-esteem, whether by saying things like, "I'm dumb," or through self-degrading behavior, know first that a longer, more expansive healing process will be needed to overcome his/her self-esteem concerns. That process, of course, will depend on your child's specific challenges and past experience, as well as his/her age, and more.

Remember to always tap on yourself first so that you can be fully present with your child. That supportive, loving presence will be enormously beneficial to your child's self-esteem over time.

If your child is willing to try Tapping with you, the best place to start is by focusing on releasing stress and relaxing the body.

Begin by asking your child how his/her body feels when s/he feels badly about him/herself, or says things like, "I'm dumb" or other expressions. Does s/he experience tension, clenching, pain, numbness or an experience of "nothingness"?

Ask your child to rate that feeling, either on a scale of 0 to 10 or using the "this much" method of measurement.

As always, use your child's words and experience as you tap with him/her.

Take a deep breath together and begin by Tapping 3 times on the Karate Chop point.

Karate Chop *(Repeat 3 times):* Even though I feel <feeling here> in my body, I'm going to be okay.

Eyebrow: This feeling in my body

Side of Eye: I feel like it'll never go away

Under Eye: This feeling in my body

Under Nose: I feel it now

Under Mouth: I don't know if it'll ever go away

Collarbone: I don't think I can get rid of this feeling

Under Arm: It's too real

Top of Head: This feeling in my body

Eyebrow: It comes up when I'm feeling badly about myself

Side of Eye: I'm not feeling good about myself right now

Under Eye: And I have this feeling in my body

Under Nose: It's okay to feel these ways

Under Mouth: They're feelings

Collarbone: They feel so real

Under Arm: But they can come and go

Top of Head: They don't have to stay with me forever

Eyebrow: I can feel calmer now

Side of Eye: I can let go of these feelings

Under Eye: I can let myself relax

Under Nose: I can trust that these feelings will go away

Under Mouth: I can relax my body now

Collarbone: I can let these feelings pass

Under Arm: It's safe to let go of these feelings now

Top of Head: Letting myself relax and feel better now

Take a deep breath together, and check back in with your child on how s/he is feeling now. If your child is willing to talk further about his/her experience, feelings, or other, do your best to listen without judgment. As always, if your child voices anything that upsets you, try not to react in the moment. Instead, take time to tap through your emotions on your own first. Once you've released your own experience, you'll be better able to be present with your child, even when s/he is resisting you.

As you navigate these issues on your own and with your child, remember that parenting, like growing up, is an ongoing process. You don't ever have to do it perfectly to be a wonderful, loving parent to your child.

Shame, Disordered Eating, Mood Disorder & Self-Loathing

When allowed to thrive in darkness, shame can literally and figuratively take over a child's life. That had been true for Tara, who, at 16 years old, was suffering from a mood disorder as well as disordered eating. Having attempted suicide more than once, she often felt overwhelmed by her critical voice, and resorted to cutting herself. For Tara, bleeding was preferable to feeling worthless and unlovable.

While meeting with a school counselor one day, Tara agreed to try Tapping. Within a few rounds, the intensity of her shame decreased from a 9 out of 10 to a 2 out of 10. From that point forward, she continually used Tapping whenever feelings of shame and worthlessness arose. Within a matter of weeks, she stopped cutting herself and was making noticeable progress with overcoming her shame.

In spite of these improvements, however, Tara continued to struggle with food, often gagging as she ate. The thought of food going into her body caused tremendous anxiety. Concerned about her health, her counselor suggested they use Tapping on her gagging reflex.

Over the course of one extended session, Tara tapped while imagining food going into her body. As she tapped, Tara visualized herself gagging on her food and then calming her body down so it could accept much-needed nourishment.

After that one Tapping session, Tara no longer struggled with gagging, and was able to begin eating regularly again for the first time in years.

Since then, Tara has been accepted into college, and continues to use Tapping on stress. She is able to eat healthfully now, and seems to be thriving on all levels.

Tara's amazing and inspiring transformation is a testament to the power of Tapping. In my years working with people who suffer from similarly toxic shame, I've noticed an interesting trend. While shame often runs deep and feels dangerously intense, it can also fade surprisingly quickly once it's successfully exposed to light. Thankfully, once shame begins to fade, all of the dangerous behaviors it promotes—cutting, disordered eating, and much more—naturally lose their appeal.

With that said, children who have adopted dangerous behaviors as a result of shame also need to understand that it takes time to create new neural pathways that support positive, healthy choices. That's why I always love to hear that people continue to use Tapping on a regular basis. By doing so, Tara will be far better equipped to adjust to college, as well as other challenges that may lie ahead.

Due to the complexity of these feelings, it is recommended, when possible, to seek out a professional who can guide your child through a deeper, more comprehensive trauma-healing process. For a list of Certified EFT practitioners, visit http://thetappingsolution.com/eft-practitioners/.

Child/Teenager Tapping: Feeling Safe with Shame

Since shame thrives in darkness, and feeling shame is a painful experience that people understandably avoid, the first step toward healing shame is Tapping on creating a sense of safety around feeling it.

To begin, ask your child to rate how much s/he doesn't want to feel or look at the shame s/he feels, either on a scale of 0 to 10 or using the "this much" method of measurement.

Take a deep breath, and begin by Tapping 3 times on the Karate Chop point.

Karate Chop *(Repeat 3 times)*: Even though I don't want to feel this shame because it's too painful and too all-consuming, I can relax now.

Eyebrow: All this shame

Side of Eye: This deep, burning shame

Under Eye: It hurts

Under Nose: I can't let myself feel it

Under Mouth: It's overwhelming

Collarbone: It's too much

Under Arm: Too dark

Top of Head: Too big

Eyebrow: It might swallow me whole

Side of Eye: But it won't go away

Under Eye: It's safe to let myself feel it now

Under Nose: It's safe to feel it now

Under Mouth: This burning shame

Collarbone: It hurts me

Under Arm: It's safe to feel it now

Top of Head: And it's safe to let it go

Eyebrow: I can let go of this shame

Side of Eye: I don't have to fear this shame

Under Eye: I can let this shame go

Under Nose: I don't need to avoid or hold onto this shame

Under Mouth: It's safe to let it go now

Collarbone: I'm safe releasing this shame

Under Arm: I'm safe without this shame

Top of Head: Letting myself relax as I release this shame now

Take a deep breath together and check back in with your child on his/her willingness to feel shame. Keep Tapping until s/he gets the desired relief.

Child Tapping: Releasing Self-Shaming Beliefs

If your child is suffering from shame, s/he likely holds beliefs around being worthless, unlovable, not good enough or something similar.

Note: If your child feels shame as a result of trauma, whether that trauma was abuse or something else, refer to the "Big T Trauma" or "Little t Trauma" section for more information about how to use Tapping to embark on a healing process (Chapter 14).

First ask your child to rate the intensity of his/her shame-fueled belief. For instance, if your child believes that "I am worthless and unlovable," ask him/her to rate how true that belief feels on a scale of 0 to 10 or using the "this much" method of measurement.

Reminder! If you're struggling with hearing your child voice his/her beliefs, be sure to tap on releasing your own reaction(s) first, before Tapping with your child.

Take a deep breath and begin by Tapping 3 times on the Karate Chop point.

Karate Chop *(Repeat 3 times)*: Even though I have this belief that I'm worthless and unlovable, I'm okay and I accept how I feel.

Eyebrow: This belief

Side of Eye: I feel worthless and unlovable

Under Eye: It hurts so badly

Under Nose: This belief

Under Mouth: It feels so true

Collarbone: And that hurts so badly

Under Arm: It's safe to feel this shame

Top of Head: Even though it hurts to feel it

Eyebrow: I'm safe letting myself feel this shame

Side of Eye: I'm safe looking at this belief

Under Eye: I'm worthless and unlovable

Under Nose: I'm worthless and unlovable

Under Mouth: Is that really true?

Collarbone: It feels so true

Under Arm: It hurts so badly

Top of Head: Is it really true?

Eyebrow: I'm safe letting myself feel this

Side of Eye: I'm safe letting this belief go now

Under Eye: It feels true sometimes

Under Nose: But is it really true?

Under Mouth: It's safe to let go of this belief now

Collarbone: It's safe to relax as I let go of this belief

Under Arm: It's safe to relax and feel love for myself

Top of Head: Letting myself feel safe as I release this belief now

Take a deep breath together and check back in with your child on how true his/her belief feels now. Keep Tapping until s/he gets the desired relief.

Since deeply rooted, limiting beliefs can take time to overwrite, encourage your child to use Tapping whenever challenging emotions and beliefs arise.

Child/Teenager Tapping: Feeling Self-Love

As your child continues to tap on releasing shame, it's helpful also to point them toward self-love and self-acceptance. Again, this is a process; and as always, if you feel you have work to do in learning to love and accept yourself, make sure to do your own Tapping as well.

Begin by asking your child to think of one thing s/he loves about him/herself. It could be her long fingers, his drawing ability, her swimming skills or his love of music. It doesn't matter what it is, as long as it's something your child can love and appreciate about him/herself.

Next ask your child to focus on that trait or skill that s/he loves and begin by Tapping on the Karate Chop point 3 times.

Karate Chop *(Repeat 3 times)*: Even though I can only love and appreciate this one thing about myself, I'm cool.

Eyebrow: This is the only thing I can love about myself

Side of Eye: There's nothing else I can love

Under Eye: The rest is shameful

Under Nose: I can't love the rest of myself

Under Mouth: I do love this one part of myself, though

Collarbone: That's it, though

Under Arm: That's all I can love about myself

Top of Head: There's nothing else about me to love

Eyebrow: I do love this one part, though

Side of Eye: I appreciate this one thing about myself

Under Eye: It's almost impressive, actually

Under Nose: I love this one thing about myself

Under Mouth: I can focus on that love now

Collarbone: I can feel that love in my mind and body now

Under Arm: Maybe I can let this love grow

Top of Head: I can love this one thing about myself even more

Eyebrow: I'm still not sure about the rest of me

Side of Eye: It still feels shameful

Under Eye: It's safe to love this one part of me, though

Under Nose: It's safe to let this loving feeling grow

Under Mouth: It's safe to feel safe now

Collarbone: I can let this love grow

Under Arm: It's safe to let myself feel loved now

Top of Head: It's safe to let this love keep growing and growing

Take a deep breath together and check back in with your child on how much love s/he can now feel for him/herself now. Keep Tapping until s/he gets the desired relief.

Child/Teenager Tapping: **Envisioning Unconditional Love**

As your child taps on releasing shame, it can also be helpful to have them tap while imagining receiving unconditional love.

Begin by asking your child to think about receiving unconditional love and acceptance. Next have him/her rate how worthy s/he feels around receiving it, either on a scale of 0 to 10 or using the "this much" method of measurement.

Take a deep breath, and begin by Tapping 3 times on the Karate Chop point.

Karate Chop *(Repeat 3 times)*: Even though I'm not sure I'm worthy of unconditional love and acceptance, I'm okay.

Eyebrow: Unconditional love

Side of Eye: Unconditional acceptance

Under Eye: I don't feel worthy

Under Nose: I'm not good enough

Under Mouth: Unconditional love

Collarbone: Unconditional acceptance

Under Arm: I'll never have that

Top of Head: I'm not worthy

Eyebrow: Is that really true?

Side of Eye: It feels true

Under Eye: There are things I appreciate about myself

Under Nose: Things I can maybe love

Under Mouth: Maybe I am worthy

Collarbone: Even if I don't always feel that I am

Under Arm: It's safe to feel worthy

Top of Head: It's safe to trust I am good enough

Eyebrow: I can believe in unconditional love

Side of Eye: I can feel worthy of receiving it

Under Eye: It's safe to imagine my life with it

Under Nose: It's safe to trust I'm worthy of unconditional love

Under Mouth: I can feel accepted and loved

Collarbone: Even if it's not always comfortable for me

Under Arm: It's safe to trust that I'm worthy of unconditional love

Top of Head: It's safe to let myself imagine receiving unconditional love now

Take a deep breath together and check back in with your child about how worthy s/he feels of receiving unconditional love now.

As you both continue Tapping through the points, ask your child to imagine, either out loud or silently in his/her mind, what it would feel, look and be like to know, without a doubt, that s/he is loved unconditionally.

As s/he taps, if it's helpful, you can gently ask questions like:

- How would you feel when you first woke up if you knew you were unconditionally loved?

- How would you feel in your body knowing you were unconditionally loved?

- What feelings of safety and security would you feel?

- If you knew for sure that you were unconditionally loved, what fears and worries could you let go of?

As you continue Tapping, encourage your child to continue imagining what s/he would feel like in his/her daily life if she felt worthy of unconditional love.

Keep Tapping through these visions for as long as your child is willing.

Exercises like these may take practice to feel real and authentic, so repeat them as often as your child is willing.

Chapter 11

Stress, Anxiety and Their Side Effects

TAPPING WITH YOUR CHILD: ANXIETY DISORDERS

Thanks to Tapping, many people find that anxiety disorders are easier to manage. Regular Tapping can lead to reduced medication, improved confidence and a better ability to adjust to new and different situations.

Before we look at using Tapping on your child's anxiety disorder, let's do some Tapping first on your experience.

Adult Tapping: Releasing Anxiety about Your Child's Disorder

When your child has an anxiety disorder, you may find yourself needing to be hypervigilant, always anticipating challenging situations. That additional effort, however important, can cause you to feel extra stress. Let's do some Tapping now on letting go of that stress so you can be more present when you tap with your child.

To begin, imagine a situation that is likely to cause your child's anxiety to magnify. Does that cause *you* to feel anxious, full of dread or just plain exhausted? Rate your own emotional response to this imagined situation on a scale of 0 to 10.

Take a deep breath, and let's begin by Tapping 3 times on the Karate Chop point:

Karate Chop *(Repeat 3 times)*: Even though it's always so stressful trying to anticipate my child's anxiety, I love myself and accept how I feel.

Eyebrow: All this stress

Side of Eye: All this energy

Under Eye: Always trying to protect my child from their anxiety

Under Nose: Always anticipating challenges they'll face

Under Mouth: All this anxiety about trying to protect them

Collarbone: It's exhausting sometimes

Under Arm: So much anxiety about their anxiety

Top of Head: It takes so much energy

Eyebrow: So much anxiety about my child's anxiety

Side of Eye: It's exhausting

Under Eye: So much anxiety

Under Nose: Letting myself feel it now

Under Mouth: And letting it all go

Collarbone: Letting myself feel it now

Under Arm: And letting it all go

Top of Head: I can release this stress from my mind and body

Eyebrow: I can trust that it will all work out

Side of Eye: It's so stressful sometimes

Under Eye: But I can let that stress go now

Under Nose: Releasing this stress from my mind and body now

Under Mouth: Letting myself relax

Collarbone: Feeling quiet and calm

Under Arm: Allowing my mind and body to relax fully now

Top of Head: Feeling peace in mind and body now

Take another deep breath, and rate the stress you feel about your child's anxiety on a scale of 0 to 10. Continue Tapping until you get the desired relief.

Now that you've had an experience, let's look at how to use Tapping with your child on their anxiety disorder.

Note: As always, when Tapping with your child, tailor your words to your child's age and experience.

QUIETING SOCIAL ANXIETY

Ryan had been struggling academically and socially since starting his second year of middle school. Noticing his distress, his mother asked if he'd be willing to tap with her one day. Although reluctant, he eventually agreed to try it.

While Tapping, Ryan shared that several kids had been teasing him during lunchtime. They tapped through how that teasing made him feel, and then again on some of the times when he'd felt ostracized. After several rounds, he relaxed noticeably.

In the days that followed, his mom noticed that he was coming home from school in a much better mood.

Over the following weeks, Ryan and his mom continued to tap together. As those weeks turned into months, his grades improved. He also found several "lunch buddies" at school. All of it together changed his entire experience at school.

This story is such a great example of how powerful Tapping is at alleviating the intense social pressures children often face at school, pressures which can be particularly intense once they reach middle school. Thanks to the Tapping he did with his mom, Ryan no longer dreaded going to school. In fact, he began to thrive on all levels. What a difference!

Child Tapping: Overcoming Social Anxiety

It's best to tap on specific situations or scenarios, so choose a social situation or scenario that your child can imagine or remember.

Next, ask your child to rate how anxious—or icky, nervous etc.—they feel when they think of it, either on a scale of 0 to 10 or by extending their arms to each side, showing their anxiety on a "this much" scale.

Then begin Tapping:

Karate Chop *(Repeat 3 times)*: Even though I feel nervous when I think about <situation here>, I'm great!

Eyebrow: So nervous/anxious

Side of Eye: I don't like feeling this way

Under Eye: Makes me feel awful inside

Under Nose: I don't like it

Under Mouth: What if they don't like me?

Collarbone: What if they tease me?

Under Arm: So nervous

Top of Head: That's okay

Eyebrow: I'm great!

Side of Eye: And everything's okay

Under Eye: I'm great!

Under Nose: I don't need to worry

Under Mouth: I'm awesome!

Collarbone: People like me

Under Arm: I can relax now

Top of Head: I'm great!

Eyebrow: I can have fun

Side of Eye: I can feel good

Under Eye: I'm great!

Under Nose: And everything's okay

Under Mouth: I can feel happy inside now

Collarbone: I can feel calm inside now

Under Arm: I'm great!

Top of Head: And everything's okay

Again have them rate their anxiety on a scale of 0 to 10, or using the "this much" method of measurement. Keep Tapping until they get the desired relief.

BEING LEFT OUT OF THE GAME

Mark, 11 years old, had been struggling with social anxiety for years. Diagnosed with Kabuki Syndrome (a rare multisystem disorder) he often felt overwhelmed by large groups, including family and people he already knew. Historically, he'd also had a difficult time adjusting to new social situations. For years his default coping mechanism had been to shut down. Once that happened, it typically took a long time for him to return to normal functioning.

Hoping to ease his intense anxiety, his mother, Rose, had introduced him to Tapping in the last years of elementary school. Thankfully, Mark had responded positively. Each time they used it, he was able to release his anxiety and relax into whatever he was doing.

One evening, Rose took Mark and her older son to a friend's house for dinner. Her friend had two children of her own, and Rose was hoping that Mark would be willing to play with them. When they arrived, he did join the group.

Before long, however, the two older boys began making a point of excluding Mark from their game. Mark's usual response to that type of situation was to

231

yell, scream and cry. Often he would get so worked up that he'd begin hitting himself. Once that happened, it would take hours before he could be calm again.

This time, however, Mark quietly came upstairs to find Rose, tapped her on the arm and whispered in her ear that he was feeling frustrated and wanted to go do some Tapping in the bathroom. Thrilled at his request, Rose jumped up and followed him. Once in the bathroom where no one could see, they started Tapping using statements like, "Even though they're leaving me out of the game, I'm a really cool kid and I'm okay!"

After a few rounds, Mark was noticeably calmer. His body relaxed, his fists weren't clenched anymore and he was smiling. He looked at Rose and told her he felt ready to go back and play with the other kids. He gave her a big hug and a high five coupled with an excited, "Thanks, Mom!" Everyone had a great time for the rest of the evening.

For years, Rose had been unsure whether Mark would ever be able to regulate his own emotions. Seeing him take charge of the situation and seek Rose out to do Tapping when he needed it was more progress than she'd dared to hope for.

As exciting as that evening was, though, it's not the end of the story. In addition to social gatherings, Tapping also became an important part of Mark's school experience. Thanks to Tapping, in fact, Mark successfully started attending a middle school with over 1,600 kids. This was huge progress compared to 4th and 5th grades, when he'd often come home from school crying, overwhelmed by frustration about homework, how much he hated school and how "stupid" he felt he was.

On the days when Mark was willing, he and Rose would do some Tapping, with Rose doing the Tapping on the points for him. As often as possible, Rose made a point of using Mark's words, which were often phrases like, "Even though I can't do this stupid homework, I'm a really cool kid and I'm okay!" Moving through the other Tapping points, they might then say, "This stupid homework… I can't do this stupid homework… homework is stupid… I'm stupid… I hate homework."

Nearly every time, Mark's entire body would relax after a few rounds. They would then take a deep breath together and she'd ask him how he felt. After another round or two, they'd finish with one final round of positive Tapping, using phrasing like: "I'm a smart kid... I can do this... homework isn't so bad... I'll finish my homework easily."

Within a matter of minutes, Mark's entire mood and demeanor would become noticeably calmer. Easily able to focus, Mark would then complete his homework. Rose was always amazed by, and incredibly grateful for, their brief moments of Tapping together.

Now that he was in a massive middle school, Mark had also made great progress with the support of his special education team. When we last emailed, in fact, Mark had asked Rose to teach Tapping to his new teacher. Determined to support him in every possible way, Rose was in the process of setting up a meeting to discuss it.

This is one of my favorite stories, not just because of the results Mark has with Tapping, but also because of how much Tapping empowers him to take control of his anxiety and his experience with other kids. Over time, as he continues to use Tapping, he will continue to realize the power he has over his own experience. That's a lesson every child, with or without Kabuki Syndrome, can use to thrive in every area of life. Amazing!

Child Tapping: Releasing Anxiety from Being Excluded

If your child is struggling with being left out of a social situation, their immediate emotional response is likely to be anger, frustration and/or sadness. If they're willing to share how they're feeling, use their words as the focus of your Tapping.

Begin by measuring the intensity of their emotional response, either on a scale of 0 to 10 or using the "this much" method of measurement.

Then begin by Tapping 3 times on the Karate Chop point:

Karate Chop *(Repeat 3 times)*: Even though I feel bad about being left out, I'm a great kid and I'm okay!

Eyebrow: I don't like being left out

Side of Eye: It makes me feel bad

Under Eye: Feeling sad about being left out

Under Nose: So sad about being left out

Under Mouth: I don't like being left out

Collarbone: It makes me mad

Under Arm: That's okay

Top of Head: I'm an awesome kid!

Eyebrow: I wasn't happy about being left out

Side of Eye: It made me feel bad

Under Eye: But I'm a great kid!

Under Nose: And people like me

Under Mouth: I can have fun when I want to

Collarbone: I'm a great kid!

Under Arm: I can play and have fun anyway

Top of Head: I can play with other kids

Eyebrow: I can have fun when I want to

Side of Eye: I'm a great kid!

Under Eye: And everything's okay

Under Nose: I can go have fun now

Under Mouth: I'm an awesome kid

Collarbone: I can have fun when I want to

Under Arm: I'm a great kid!

Top of Head: And everything's okay

Ask your child to measure the intensity of his or her feelings about being left out now, either on a scale of 0 to 10 or using the "this much" method of measurement. Keep Tapping until s/he gets the desired relief.

QUIETING A PANIC ATTACK

One of the great things about teaching Tapping to children is how much it empowers them to help themselves as well as their peers. This story was recently sent to me by the mother of a college student and athlete. It's a great example of how powerful Tapping is for suppressing panic attacks.

Tanya, 20 years old, is a college student who runs cross-country races. Since learning Tapping from her mom a few years ago, she's used it to quiet the anxiety she sometimes feels, whether about her running, studies, or other.

On the phone with her mom one day, Tanya shared a story about a cross-country teammate who began suffering from a panic attack in the middle of a practice run. Tanya stopped next to her teammate, and told her friend, "Just do what I do," as she began Tapping through the points.

Neither Tanya nor her teammate spoke a word. Instead, they tapped through the points. After two rounds of Tapping, her teammate's panic attacked had ended, and they were both able to resume their run. Tanya was thrilled to be able to help her teammate in this way.

Panic attacks tend to feel overwhelming, physically as well as emotionally, so the most important thing is to start Tapping. As Tanya did with her friend, have your child follow along and tap through the points with you. Let them know they can speak if they choose to, but they don't have to.

Once the panic attack is over, if your child is open to it, you can try talking to them about their panic response. Ask them to continue Tapping through the points as they answer questions like:

- What did you feel in your body when the panic attack was happening?
- What do you feel in your body now?
- What caused your panic?
- Is there anything else you'd like to share?

As always, respect your child's boundaries and don't push them to address anything they're not ready or willing to discuss. If they're not interested in talking, tap with them in silence for as long as they want you to.

MANAGING OBSESSIVE BEHAVIOR

When faced with overwhelming anxiety, some kids may resort to obsessive behavior. Whether classified as OCD, impulse control disorder, or something else, these behaviors often involve ritualized movement. Tapping can be enormously helpful in these cases, as it gives children a healthy way to release anxiety while doing what they're naturally inclined to do—move their body.

This story about Jenna's 5-year-old son, David, is a great example of how effective Tapping can be for OCD.

Jenna and her family had recently moved to a new town, which meant David had to attend a new elementary school. In the early weeks after their move, Jenna had to live apart from her family, as her work required her to be several hundred miles away.

Clearly struggling with the stress and anxiety of so many big changes happening at once, David began suffering from Trichotillomania, an impulse control disorder (which some consider to be correlated with OCD) that involves obsessively pulling out your own eyelashes.

Once Jenna's work allowed her to return to her family, she began Tapping on David. Addressing his perceived need to pull out his eyelashes, as well as his intense anxiety over their move and temporarily disjointed family life, David was able to relax and begin making a healthier adjustment to his new home.

After only a few days of intermittent Tapping, David's Trichotillomania disappeared.

Child Tapping: Overcoming Obsessive Behavior

Similar to panic attacks, the goal here is to *do* the Tapping. Whether you tap on your child or they tap along with you, the most important thing to do is quiet the stress response that's causing your child's obsessive behavior.

You don't have to talk while you tap, but if you think it would help your child, you can use some general positive Tapping phrases like:

Karate Chop *(Repeat 3 times)*: Even though I feel like I have to do this behavior, and I can't stop it, I'm a great kid and I'm okay.

Eyebrow: I have to do this

Side of Eye: I can't stop it

Under Eye: I have to do this

Under Nose: It helps me

Under Mouth: That's okay

Collarbone: I'm a great kid

Under Arm: And I'm okay

Top of Head: It's safe to focus on Tapping for a minute

Eyebrow: I can feel safe and tap for a bit

Side of Eye: It's safe to let myself relax

Under Eye: I'm a great kid

Under Nose: And I'm okay

Under Mouth: I'm great just as I am

Collarbone: I can do this Tapping thing

Under Arm: I can feel safe doing this Tapping

Top of Head: It's safe to feel safe now

Eyebrow: I can let myself relax a bit

Side of Eye: I can feel safe Tapping

Under Eye: I'm a great kid

Under Nose: And I'm okay

Under Mouth: I can feel quiet in my body now

Collarbone: I can feel calm in my body now

Under Arm: Feeling calm and safe in my body now

Top of Head: I'm a great kid and I'm okay

Keep Tapping until your child gets the desired relief. While some children may overcome obsessive behavior quickly, others may need more time. Whatever you do, continue Tapping!

Child Tapping: Overcoming Selective Mutism

In some cases children feel so overwhelmed by anxiety that they feel unable to talk. Again, the best course of action is to start Tapping.

The only caveat here is not to make the "goal" of your Tapping be the talking. Instead, let your child know that s/he doesn't have to talk at any point, and give them the space and time they need to overcome the selective mutism on their own terms and timeline. (And if that makes you anxious, make sure to do your own Tapping on how *you're* feeling.)

To begin, simply have your child follow along as you tap through the points (or tap on the points for them).

If your child is okay with you speaking while you both tap, you can try saying positive phrases as you tap through the points:

Karate Chop *(Repeat 3 times)*: Even though I don't want to talk, I'm a great kid and I'm okay.

Eyebrow: I won't talk

Side of Eye: I can't talk

Under Eye: It doesn't feel safe to talk right now

Under Nose: It's too much

Under Mouth: And I can't talk right now

Collarbone: I don't want to talk

Under Arm: That's okay

Top of Head: I'm a great kid

Eyebrow: And I'm okay

Side of Eye: I don't have to talk

Under Eye: I can be quiet

Under Nose: And I can feel safe in my body

Under Mouth: I don't have to talk

Collarbone: I can talk when I'm ready

Under Arm: I can feel safe not talking

Top of Head: And I can feel safe talking

Eyebrow: It's okay if I don't want to talk

Side of Eye: I'm a great kid!

Under Eye: I can talk when I feel like it

Under Nose: I can feel safe being quiet

Under Mouth: I can feel safe talking when I'm ready

Collarbone: I'm a great kid!

Under Arm: And I'm okay

Top of Head: It's safe to feel safe and calm now

Keep Tapping for as long as your child is willing or until s/he gets the desired relief.

TAPPING WITH YOUR CHILD: SLEEP

Kids often struggle with sleep for similar reasons as adults. They may be anxious, overwhelmed by the events of the day, over-stimulated before bed, or they may struggle to quiet their mind and body for other reasons. Children may also experience physical discomfort or pain, or feel afraid of the dark or certain noises.

Fortunately even a few minutes of Tapping at bedtime, especially when it's done consistently, can quickly resolve sleep issues and allow children (as well as their parents!) to get restful, restorative sleep on a regular basis.

As anyone who has ever struggled with sleep knows, that kind of consistent improvement is life-changing.

The best first step, however, is using Tapping before bed to improve your own sleep. If you tend to wake up tired or experience other sleep challenges, your child may pick up on that and fall into similar patterns.

Once we look at how you can use Tapping at bedtime yourself, we'll look at how to tap with your child on improving his/her sleep.

Adult Tapping: Falling Asleep, Waking Rested

There are so many reasons we struggle with getting restorative sleep on a regular basis. Some people wake up throughout the night or wake up tired without knowing why. Others may struggle with falling asleep during the week when they travel or when schedules change.

In this Tapping script we'll focus on relaxing when it's time to fall asleep. Even if that's not your particular issue around sleep, I urge you to try Tapping at bedtime, using this script or simply Tapping on what you're feeling or experiencing in your body.

By regularly using Tapping to quiet your mind and body before sleep, you're more likely to wake up feeling rested and energized.

Since our goal is to quiet the mind, we'll skip the rating step, and begin with a deep breath.

Next, let's begin by Tapping 3 times on the Karate Chop point:

Karate Chop *(Repeat 3 times)*: Even though I'm not yet relaxed enough to fall asleep, I love myself and accept how I feel.

Eyebrow: It's time to sleep

Side of Eye: My mind won't stop buzzing

Under Eye: And my body feels tense

Under Nose: I need to relax

Under Mouth: But I don't know how

Collarbone: My mind won't stop going

Under Arm: And my body won't relax

Top of Head: It's time to get some sleep

Eyebrow: But it's hard to quiet the mental noise

Side of Eye: And relax my body

Under Eye: That's okay

Under Nose: I can let go of this pattern

Under Mouth: I can quiet my mind and body

Collarbone: I can let go of these busy thoughts

Under Arm: I can relax my body

Top of Head: Release any pain or discomfort I feel in my body now

Eyebrow: Allowing my body to relax and feel calm now

Side of Eye: Releasing any stress I may be feeling

Under Eye: Letting go of whatever happened today

Under Nose: And releasing tomorrow, too

Under Mouth: Quieting my mind and body now

Collarbone: Allowing myself to feel quiet and comfortable now

Under Arm: Feeling complete peace and quiet in mind and body now

Top of Head: Fully relaxing my mind and body now

Take a deep breath.

Keep Tapping if you'd like, and know that you can return to this Tapping meditation as often as you'd like.

Now that you've had an experience, let's look at how to use Tapping with your child to improve his/her sleep.

Note: As always, when Tapping with your child, tailor your words to your child's age and experience.

RELEASING STRESS, SLEEPING SOUNDLY

Nine-year-old Becca had been struggling for years with sleeping through the night, and would frequently wake her parents in the early morning hours. It had been an exhausting pattern her parents had long hoped would stop. The years had ticked by, however, and still, a full night's rest was a rare treat.

At bedtime on the second night of a new school year, Becca suddenly burst into tears. She shared with her parents how overwhelmed she was feeling about starting in a new grade. Hoping to help her relax, they led her through several rounds of Tapping on how she was feeling.

Within a matter of minutes, Becca visibly calmed down and immediately fell fast asleep. Just as important, she stayed asleep the entire night.

From that night onward, Becca's parents made sure to do a few minutes of Tapping with her at bedtime. She now sleeps through the night regularly.

Just those few minutes of Tapping on releasing the stress of her day completely transformed her and her parents' sleep. Wow!

Child Tapping: Quieting an Active Mind at Bedtime

Before doing general Tapping on relaxing and calming down at bedtime, it's a good idea to find out if there's anything your child needs to talk about first.

As one example, a friend of mine learned one day that her son, who's often surrounded by friends, had been left out during recess at school. Once he'd released his anger and sadness about being rejected, he fell asleep immediately, and woke up happy and excited for school.

This same pattern can happen if your child is feeling over-stimulated at bedtime, which can be caused by being excited about an upcoming event, watching a movie, or something else.

To begin, have your child tap through the points as you ask him or her:

- Is there anything you want to talk about that would help you feel calmer?

- Is there anything that happened today that you want to tap on?

- Is there anything we can talk about that might help you feel ready to sleep?

If there is, let your child talk through it as you tap on or with him or her.

Once s/he has let go of whatever was on her or his mind, if s/he is not yet ready to fall asleep, you can do some general Tapping.

Child Tapping: Relaxing Body & Mind at Bedtime

Since the goal is to fall asleep, we'll skip the rating step and go straight to Tapping 3 times on the Karate Chop point:

Karate Chop *(Repeat 3 times)*: Even though it's bedtime and I'm not sure I'm ready to sleep yet, I'm a great kid and I'm okay.

Eyebrow: Not sure I'm ready to sleep

Side of Eye: But it's my bedtime

Under Eye: Not sure I'm ready to sleep

Under Nose: That's okay

Under Mouth: I'm a great kid!

Collarbone: I can feel quiet now

Under Arm: I can feel calm now

Top of Head: Feeling calm and quiet now

Eyebrow: Time to sleep

Side of Eye: Sleep feels good!

Under Eye: Time to sleep

Under Nose: Feeling calm and quiet now

Under Mouth: Letting myself drift off to sleep

Collarbone: To dream happy dreams

Under Arm: Relaxing my body now

Top of Head: Feeling quiet all over

Eyebrow: Feeling calm

Side of Eye: Ready to sleep

Under Eye: Feeling calm and quiet now

Under Nose: I can go to sleep easily now

Under Mouth: Letting myself go to sleep

Collarbone: Feeling calm and quiet

Under Arm: Ready to sleep now

Top of Head: Ready to sleep now

Keep Tapping until your child is ready to sleep or already asleep.

Child Tapping: Falling Back Asleep

While Tapping can't guarantee that your child will never wake up earlier than you'd like, it can help your child to fall back asleep when s/he has been awoken by a noise or other disruption.

Since the goal is to fall back asleep, we'll again go straight to Tapping 3 times on the Karate Chop point:

Karate Chop *(Repeat 3 times)*: Even though I was woken up and I'm not sure I'll be able to go back to sleep, I'm a great kid and I'm okay.

Eyebrow: Not sure I'll be able to go back to sleep

Side of Eye: But it's still nighttime

Under Eye: Not sure I'll go back to sleep

Under Nose: That's okay

Under Mouth: I'm a great kid!

Collarbone: I can feel quiet now

Under Arm: I can feel calm now

Top of Head: Feeling calm and quiet now

Eyebrow: Time to sleep

Side of Eye: I can fall back asleep easily

Under Eye: I can let myself sleep again

Under Nose: Feeling calm and quiet now

Under Mouth: Letting myself drift off to sleep

Collarbone: To dream happy dreams

Under Arm: Relaxing my body now

Top of Head: Feeling quiet all over

Eyebrow: Feeling calm

Side of Eye: Ready to go back to sleep

Under Eye: Feeling calm and quiet now

Under Nose: I can fall back asleep easily now

Under Mouth: Letting myself go to sleep

Collarbone: Feeling calm and quiet

Under Arm: Ready to sleep now

Top of Head: Ready to sleep now

Keep Tapping until your child is ready to go back to sleep or already asleep.

TAPPING WITH YOUR CHILD: NIGHTMARES

At some point in their development, most children struggle with nightmares. While these bad dreams are often triggered by the normal stress of growing up, they can also result from specific events, such as watching a scary movie, being chased and more. For children who have experienced trauma, it's common to have frequent nightmares for six months or longer.

Whatever the cause, nightmares are intensely scary because the dreamer feels powerless to protect themselves and/or others. As tempting as it is to tell your child that nightmares aren't real, we know that rational thinking doesn't allay fears. Instead, you can use Tapping to help your child recreate a sense of safety, helping him/her to release fear and his/her perceived powerlessness.

Before we look at how to use Tapping with your child to resolve nightmares, however, let's first release some of the stress you may experience as a result of your child's, and likely your own, troubled sleep.

Adult Tapping: Releasing the Stress from Your Child's Nightmares

When you think about your child's nightmare(s), how much stress do you feel on a scale of 0 to 10?

Take a deep breath. We'll start by Tapping 3 times on the Karate Chop point:

Karate Chop *(Repeat 3 times)*: Even though I feel stressed about my child's nightmares, I love myself and accept how I feel.

Eyebrow: All this stress

Side of Eye: I want to stop the nightmares

Under Eye: Why is he having these nightmares?

Under Nose: All this worrying

Under Mouth: All this stress

Collarbone: I feel powerless to stop these nightmares

Under Arm: All this worrying

Top of Head: It's safe to let go of these worry thoughts now

Eyebrow: It's safe to relax

Side of Eye: These nightmares aren't my fault

Under Eye: And I can help him to stop having them

Under Nose: It's safe to feel safe now

Under Mouth: It's safe to relax now

Collarbone: Letting all this worry go now

Under Arm: Allowing myself to relax

Top of Head: It's safe to feel safe

Eyebrow: Relaxing my mind and body now

Side of Eye: I can help him to stop having these nightmares

Under Eye: I can let go of these worry thoughts

Under Nose: And release this stress

Under Mouth: Letting myself relax now

Collarbone: It's safe to feel safe

Under Arm: It's safe to relax now

Top of Head: Feeling peaceful now

Take a deep breath and check back in with the stress and worry you were feeling around your child's nightmares. On a scale of 0 to 10, how emotionally charged do they feel now? Keep Tapping until you get the desired relief.

Now that you've had an experience with Tapping, let's look at how to use Tapping with your child.

Note: As always, tailor your words to your child's age and experience.

Scary Start to Happy Ending

Patty's daughter, Kira, now 9 years old, is highly sensitive and often suffers from intense emotions and fears. For months at a time, she would cry each morning as she recalled vivid nightmares she'd had the night before. Although her parents continued to remind her that her nightmares weren't real, they didn't stop.

This pattern seemed to perpetuate itself, and it was adding enormous stress to their morning and evening routines. Desperate for a new approach, her parents tried Tapping with her at night, and often during the day as well.

They tapped with Kira on what had happened that day, how she was feeling, as well as everyday experiences ranging from school and homework to interactions with her friends and teachers. When Kira was willing, they also tapped on the anxiety and fear she was feeling around her nightmares themselves. At bedtime her parents also made sure to include some positive rounds of Tapping about sleeping soundly and having happy dreams.

After years of interrupted sleep, Kira and her parents were thrilled to find that her nightmares began dissipating soon after they began Tapping more regularly. They were all now getting a good night's sleep, and waking up happy and rested as a result.

As the weeks went by, Kira shared that although some of her dreams still start off feeling scary, they now end on a happy note. As a result, they no longer cause her to go to sleep or wake up afraid.

Plus, thanks to Tapping, everyone in the household can once again get the restorative sleep that's so essential to health and wellness.

Before we look at how to tap with your child on their nightmares, let's look at one more story. You'll notice that in both of these stories, the key to transforming dreams is empowering your child to imagine a new ending to their nightmares.

Dinosaur (or Other Big Scary Creature) Nightmares

Nearly two years had passed since Kyle had seen the larger-than-life dinosaur models in the museum, but their size still haunted him.

The models he'd seen had huge teeth and were taller than some buildings. He was scared that they would bite him; his fears frequently played themselves out in nightmares that caused him to awaken in a state of panic. He shared with Deirdre, his EFT practitioner, that once he'd even rolled out of bed during a dinosaur nightmare, and his mom had to come in to save him.

As always with Tapping, it's important to acknowledge the emotions that children are feeling. With kids, however, it's also important not to go too negative, since that can magnify the challenges that they're already facing.

To balance this out, Deirdre used setup statements like, "Even though the scary dinosaurs woke me up with a fright and I was scared, I'm a great kid and really brave and strong." As they proceeded through the rounds, she used reminders like "I choose to sleep peacefully now," and "I'm a big, strong, brave kid."

Since Kyle was most afraid of the dinosaur's size, Deirdre told him the story of the elephant who was scared by the mouse. They agreed that, since he was a big, strong, brave kid, if he ever had a nightmare again, he could ask the dinosaur to go away.

One of the highlights of this session is how Deirdre empowered Kyle. In addition to reminding him that he himself is big, strong and brave, she gave him another "weapon"—his voice—that he can use to get the dinosaurs to go away. Kyle immediately understood that he had a unique advantage—the power to use his words to protect himself.

Child Tapping: Neutralizing Nightmares and Tapping at Bedtime to Prevent Nightmares

For both Kyle and Kira, the key to resolving nightmares was using Tapping to quiet their fears and empower them with a way to protect and assert themselves. For Kira, that meant creating a new, "not scary" ending to her nightmares. For Kyle, that meant reclaiming his voice as a way of defending himself.

We'll look at several different ways to address nightmares—when your child is remembering his/her nightmare, in the middle of the night when a nightmare has woken him or her up and as a preventive measure at bedtime.

If your child is fearful about a nightmare s/he has already had...

Begin by having your child rate how scary his/her nightmare was, using with the 0 to 10 scale or the "this much" method of measurement.

Then begin Tapping, using your child's words whenever possible:

Karate Chop *(Repeat 3 times)*: Even though I had this scary nightmare, I'm a great kid and everything's okay.

Eyebrow: This scary nightmare

Side of Eye: I didn't like it

Under Eye: So scary

Under Nose: But I'm safe

Under Mouth: I'm a great kid!

Collarbone: Everything's okay now

Under Arm: I'm an awesome kid

Top of Head: And I'm safe now

Next, continue Tapping through the points as you talk to your child about imagining a better ending to the nightmare. Can s/he yell at the monster or creature to "go away"? Can s/he close a door or find a safe place in the dream?

Keep Tapping through the points as you and your child imagine better endings. With younger kids you can frame voice as his/her magic power, or have him/her imagine that s/he is faster and/or stronger than whatever is scaring her/him.

Above all, use your imagination and go with your gut. Let the story lead to an ending that soothes and comforts your child. If that doesn't work, just keep Tapping on the points until s/he feels more relaxed, and then try completing this exercise at another time.

When your child is awoken by a nightmare…

Gently let your child know you'd like to tap on him/her. If s/he is willing, begin Tapping on the points of her/his body. Since s/he is likely to feel scared and disoriented, let her/him lead the way:

- If s/he *does* want to talk about the nightmare, let her/him do that as you tap on her/him until s/he is relaxed enough to fall back asleep.

- If s/he *doesn't* want to talk about her/his nightmare, keep Tapping on as many points as you can. Don't worry if you can only get to one point. Just keep Tapping. You can also reassure her/him that s/he is safe, and everything's okay.

Tapping at bedtime to prevent nightmares...

A few minutes of Tapping at bedtime can relax your child, improve the quality of his or her sleep and decrease nightmares. The key here, though, is not to focus on your child's nightmares unless s/he wants to. Most of all, use your bedtime Tapping as a way to relax, let go of any stress or fear and get ready for a good night's sleep.

Since this is general Tapping and we don't want to get your child focused on fear or nightmares at bedtime (unless they *want* to tap on them), skip the rating step and begin Tapping through the points.

You can begin with a question like:

- Is there anything that you want to tap on?

It could be something that happened that day or just something that's on your child's mind. If s/he is willing, have her or him talk about it while Tapping through the points. When s/he is done and can talk about whatever it is with little to no emotional charge, move to the positive rounds of Tapping below.

If there's nothing your child wants to tap on, go directly to the positive round below.

Eyebrow: I'm a great kid!

Side of Eye: And I'm ready to feel calm now

Under Eye: And let go of my day

Under Nose: I can relax my body

Under Mouth: And feel quiet inside now

Collarbone: It's time to sleep

Under Arm: And have happy dreams

Top of Head: I feel calm and ready to sleep now

Keep Tapping until your child is either relaxed enough to go to sleep, or has fallen asleep.

Child Tapping: **Neutralizing Nightmares after Trauma**

Nightmares that are triggered by trauma may take longer to diffuse, though Tapping is incredibly powerful for overcoming trauma, including PTSD, in children and adults.

As always, be sure to ask your child's permission to tap. If s/he is willing, have her or him tap with you, or tap on her or him, while s/he tells the story of the nightmare.

If it takes multiple, repeated tellings to neutralize the nightmare, either in one sitting or several, don't worry. That's completely normal.

If Tapping only on his/her nightmare doesn't provide sufficient relief, you may need to tap with him/her on the trauma s/he experienced.

Note: If you were involved in the trauma that is troubling your child, be sure to use Tapping yourself before Tapping with your child. It's critical to neutralize the emotional charge you're feeling before you address your child's trauma. This way you can be fully present with your child instead of potentially adding your own emotional baggage to the situation.

When you're ready, ask your child if s/he is willing to tap on what happened. If so, ask her or him how s/he feels—afraid, angry, etc.—and then have him or her rate how intensely s/he feels it, either on a 0 to 10 scale or using the "this much" method of measurement.

If your child is willing to talk about what s/he remembers, let her or him do so as s/he taps, or you tap on her/him. Have her/him tell and retell the story until the emotional charge is gone. This may happen in one sitting or over a period of several days, weeks or months. The important thing is to keep Tapping through it until the emotional charge of that original event has dissipated.

If your child is willing to tap on what happened but doesn't want to talk, begin with general Tapping. For instance, if a child was in a car crash, you might lead him/her through rounds like this:

Karate Chop *(Repeat 3 times)*: Even though I was so scared by that car crash, I'm a great kid and I'm safe now.

Eyebrow: So scared

Side of Eye: I was so scared

Under Eye: It was so loud

Under Nose: And I was so scared

Under Mouth: So scary

Collarbone: I didn't know what was happening

Under Arm: So scary

Top of Head: All that noise

Eyebrow: It was so scary

Side of Eye: It was so fast

Under Eye: I was so scared

Under Nose: I'm safe now

Under Mouth: I was so scared

Collarbone: I'm safe now

Under Arm: I can stop being scared

Top of Head: I'm safe now

Eyebrow: I'm okay

Side of Eye: I'm safe now

Under Eye: I can stop feeling scared

Under Nose: I'm safe now

Under Mouth: Everything's okay

Collarbone: And I'm okay

Under Arm: I'm a great kid

Top of Head: And everything's okay

Have your child rate his or her emotional intensity again, and keep Tapping until the emotional charge is gone. Again, this may happen quickly, or over a longer period of time.

Chapter 12

School Issues

TAPPING WITH YOUR CHILD: PERFORMANCE ANXIETY

Children are under so much pressure these days. From academics to athletics, the arts, and any number of other extracurricular activities, there's a huge focus on measuring and tracking children's progress. Although helpful in some ways, this emphasis on performance creates an enormous amount of stress, which increases performance anxiety in children and parents alike.

Let's begin by looking at how this focus on performance is affecting our experience as parents, and then how you can use Tapping to quiet your child's performance anxiety.

Is Your Parenting Measuring Up?

With so much attention being paid to how children are performing, parents are also feeling pressured to perform in their parenting, as well. Even when our children are very young, we may notice children who are performing better than our own and begin to worry about our children and also question our worthiness as parents. We may wonder, "Why isn't my child performing as well as others? Am I reading enough with my child? Am I spending enough time practicing math, sports, and more? Am I serving the 'right' foods, making sure s/he gets the optimal amount of exercise?" The list of concerns goes on and on.

As time passes, our child's performance—at school, in sports, the arts, even on the playground and during playdates—may begin to feel like a reflection of our parenting. This creates enormous stress and anxiety that then has a profound effect on our experience around parenting, as well as on our children.

Let's do some Tapping now on releasing any anxiety you may feel around your child's performance, as well as your own parenting.

Adult Tapping: Overcoming Parental Performance Anxiety

Focus on an area where your child isn't performing as well as you'd like them to. It can be an isolated incident, like a poor test grade, or an ongoing issue.

When you think about that issue, notice the primary emotion you feel. For instance, do you feel secretly ashamed that your child isn't performing at the same level as other children? Are you scared that your child won't be adequately prepared to succeed in life? Are you worried that you don't measure up as a parent, and that your inadequacies are negatively impacting your child?

Be honest with yourself about how you feel and rate the intensity of your primary emotion on a scale of 0 to 10.

Take a deep breath. We'll start by Tapping 3 times on the Karate Chop point:

Karate Chop *(Repeat 3 times)*: Even though I'm so scared and worried about my child's performance, I love myself and accept how I feel.

Eyebrow: Why isn't s/he performing at a higher level?

Side of Eye: Is his/her schooling to blame?

Under Eye: Is there something wrong?

Under Nose: All this pressure

Under Mouth: All this worry about how my child is performing

Collarbone: What if s/he doesn't measure up?

Under Arm: What will that mean for his/her future?

Top of Head: All this worry

Eyebrow: So much stress

Side of Eye: Maybe I'm not doing enough to help him/her

Under Eye: Maybe it's my fault

Under Nose: All this worry

Under Mouth: So much stress

Collarbone: It's too much

Under Arm: It's not helping my child or me

Top of Head: It's safe to let go of this stress and anxiety

Eyebrow: It's safe to relax about my child's performance

Side of Eye: Parenting doesn't have to feel like a race

Under Eye: I can let go of this worry and stress

Under Nose: And trust that this doesn't have to feel like a race

Under Mouth: Releasing this worry about my child's performance

Collarbone: I can trust in my parenting

Under Arm: And quiet this worrying around my child's performance

Top of Head: It's safe to feel relaxed when I think about my child's performance

When you're ready, take a deep breath. When you focus on your child's performance, how intensely do you feel your primary emotion now? Rate it on a scale of 0 to 10. Continue Tapping until you get the desired relief.

Now that you've had an experience, let's look at how to tap with your child on their performance anxiety.

Note: As always, when Tapping with your child, tailor your words to your child's age and experience.

Overcoming Math Test Anxiety

Math had always been Naomi's weak point. A great student in every other subject, Naomi's math grades had been just barely above the passing mark since elementary school. Now that she was in high school and colleges would be checking her transcripts, her low math grades were becoming a bigger problem.

Given that her math scores had been low for so many years, Naomi's parents understandably assumed that math simply wasn't her strong suit. To help her improve, they found her a math tutor, hoping the extra practice would help Naomi perform better, especially on tests.

After working with Naomi, the tutor shared some surprising news. In the comfort of their home, Naomi had successfully completed all of the math exercises the tutor had given her. Rather than lacking skill or knowledge in math, the tutor suggested that Naomi might be suffering from math test anxiety.

Willing to pursue this as a possibility, Naomi's mother did some Tapping with her on how much she hated math and dreaded math tests. After this general Tapping on her anxiety about math, her mother then asked Naomi if anyone had ever laughed at her in math class. Naomi recalled a time in kindergarten, when she was 5 years old, when the other students had laughed at her for not being able to count to 100. The two of them tapped together on releasing the embarrassment she'd felt at the time. Once they were done releasing the emotional charge of that event, Naomi's mother told her to go to the bathroom before the next math test and do some Tapping in the stall to calm her anxiety.

As a result of her Tapping, Naomi's math grades increased by almost 40%. She has since attended a Math & Sciences high school, where she was often called upon to help other students who were struggling in math—and best of all, one day she came home and announced to her mother that math was her favorite subject.

This story was graciously contributed by:
http://www.eft-Tapping.learnandenjoy.com/eft-math-test-multiplication-tables-mathematics.html

Child Tapping: Releasing Test Anxiety

The best place to start with test anxiety is on the anxiety itself. Begin by asking your child to rate his or her test anxiety, either on a scale of 0 to 10 or using the "this much" method of measurement.

Then begin by Tapping 3 times on the Karate Chop point:

Karate Chop *(Repeat 3 times)*: Even though I'm so anxious about this test, I'm great and everything's okay.

Eyebrow: So anxious about this test

Side of Eye: What if I mess it up?

Under Eye: So nervous about messing it up

Under Nose: So much anxiety about taking this test

Under Mouth: All this nervousness

Collarbone: I don't want to take it

Under Arm: This test is making me so anxious

Top of Head: It feels like such a big deal

Eyebrow: So anxious about this test

Side of Eye: Is it such a big deal?

Under Eye: It's just a test!

Under Nose: I can handle this test

Under Mouth: I don't have to be so anxious

Collarbone: It's just a test

Under Arm: I can do this

Top of Head: Releasing this test anxiety now

Eyebrow: I can focus on learning

Side of Eye: And let go of this anxiety

Under Eye: It's just a test

Under Nose: I can relax and focus on practicing

Under Mouth: Letting go of this anxiety

Collarbone: I'm great!

Under Arm: And I can do this

Top of Head: Relaxing and letting this anxiety go now

Take a deep breath together and check back in with your child on his/her anxiety. Keep Tapping until s/he gets the desired relief.

If your child's test anxiety stems from a past "trigger" event, as was the case for Naomi, ask him or her to tell the story while Tapping through the points. Once s/he can repeat the entire story without experiencing an emotional charge, you know you've neutralized that original event.

Overcoming "I Hate Math!" Angst

"I'm terrible at math, and I hate it!" Macy yelled, holding up her paper to show her mom which homework page she hadn't yet completed. At 9 years old, Macy had always been thorough with her homework. This outburst wasn't her normal behavior, so her mom knew something had happened. After asking why she hated math so much, Macy shared something that had happened at school that day.

During a math exercise in class, the teacher had asked students to stand as soon as they had completed their math worksheets. All of the kids stood up before Macy. She was now convinced that she was bad at math, and shared how stupid she'd felt, being the last one to finish when all of the other students in her class were already standing.

Macy and her mother had already tapped together many times, so her mother began leading her through some Tapping rounds on her belief around being bad at math, and about feeling stupid being the last student in the class to stand.

When she checked back in with Macy on how she was feeling, Macy shared that she'd been scared that her teacher would be angry with her for finishing last, and so they did several Tapping rounds on Macy's fear that her teacher would be angry with her. Macy felt calmer, and they then finished with a couple of positive Tapping rounds on how she wanted to do her best in math, and how she could do anything if she was willing to practice.

When Macy was feeling better, her mother went through her math homework with her, and walked her through the process of adding columns together and then carrying the numbers over. Macy was open and receptive to her mother's guidance, and even agreed to complete an extra practice sheet.

Macy completed the practice sheet in record time. When she was done, her mother said, "You can stand up now." She gave her daughter a big high five. Macy was beaming with pride and excitement. She hugged her mom and exclaimed, "Mom, you're my hero!"

Needless to say, both Macy and her mom were elated at her transformation. Instead of suffering under the belief that she was bad at math, Macy quickly realized that it was her anxiety, and not her math ability, that had slowed her down in class earlier that day. Just as important, Macy now has a tool that she can use to manage her anxiety, which will enable her to realize her full potential in math and beyond.

Before we look at how to tap with your child on "I'm bad at ____" beliefs, let's look at another related story.

Resolving Homework Angst

"I raised my hand first of all to say thank you because I have been aware of Tapping for a few years now. I use it intermittently, and I have used it with my kids here and there. And since we started this group, I have been Tapping a lot more, like everybody else."

Gabrielle shared this with us all during the fourth and final call of the Parents Group program. The night before, her 9-year-old son had had a complete meltdown about his homework. This was unusual—he'd always been conscientious about completing his work, but there had been one specific section of this particular night's homework that had caused him to panic. The assignment was to write a personal mission statement.

Instead of feeding his panic, Gabrielle, who has her own coaching business, did something she'd never been able to do before. "For the first time I experienced myself as a coach with my kids...That was an interesting awareness for me," she added.

As soon as her son began his meltdown about writing a personal mission statement, she sat down on his bed with him and asked him if she could tap on him. He nodded yes, so she began Tapping through the points on his body, as she asked him about his homework.

Instead of focusing immediately on the part of his homework that he was struggling with, she asked him to go back to all the parts he'd already completed. "What were you telling yourself when you were working on those sections?" she asked him. He answered that he'd read those questions and thought, "Oh, I know that." She asked him what he said to himself when he got to the mission statement question. He said he immediately thought, "I don't know."

When Gabrielle asked him where on his body he felt that "I don't know" feeling, he pointed to a spot on one side of his head. She tapped on that point for a moment as he repeated, "I don't know" several times. Gabrielle then asked him where on his body he'd felt the "I know this one" for the previous homework questions he'd already completed. He pointed to a spot on the opposite side of his head.

"Do you think those two spots could meet in the middle somewhere?" she asked him.

He shrugged, nodding slightly. "I guess."

Gabrielle began Tapping on both sides of his head simultaneously. She asked her son to go through all of the questions he did know and talk through his answers. They continued doing this as she tapped on both sides of his head. When she could sense him beginning to relax as he talked through what he did know, she began Tapping the two fingers toward each other until they met in a mid-point spot.

After just a few minutes of Tapping, his entire energy shifted. He went right to work on his personal mission statement and even enjoyed writing it. Thanks to Tapping, his meltdown had morphed into inspiration.

Imagine what would happen if more parents tapped on their kids while they did homework! Their entire experience around learning could be transformed.

As excited as I was about Gabrielle's bold spirit when it came to Tapping with her kids, I was also moved by her reflections about it. "Tapping is reminding me to become present with my kids and actually be in that moment," she explained. "I am currently trying to build my coaching business, and so a lot of the time my head is there instead of with my kids. I am thinking, *I just have to get through this dinnertime or this bedtime, and then I can get back to work.* So with Tapping I am just going, *Hey, I see this issue and I have got this tool at my fingertips. So cool, let's just start doing it.*"

Gabrielle explained that since the group started, she'd focused most of her Tapping on "I am" statements, which are her beliefs about herself, her life and what's possible for her. It had been freeing up a lot of her energy, and she'd never felt so powerful as a mother or as a coach. The timing was perfect, too, as she'd recently left her husband and initiated divorce proceedings. As a result, she was feeling a lot of pressure to grow her coaching business. She'd always done her coaching when she could fit it in, but now needed to make it a higher priority. Tapping on her beliefs about herself had upped her game as a coach and as a mom.

Child Tapping: Transforming "I'm Bad at _____" Beliefs

If you hear your child claiming they're "bad at" a skill or subject, or that they "can't do" something, as always, ask first if they're willing to do some Tapping on it. If they agree, have them rate how true it feels, either on a scale of 0 to 10 or using the "this much" method of measurement.

Then, if you can, ask them:

- Why do you think you're <state belief>?
- Where in your body do you feel it?

Then begin by Tapping 3 times on the Karate Chop point. For Gabrielle's son, that might look something like:

Karate Chop *(Repeat 3 times)*: Even though I keep telling myself I don't know this, I'm an awesome kid and everything's okay!

Eyebrow: I don't know

Side of Eye: I can't answer this question

Under Eye: I don't know how

Under Nose: I hate this question

Under Mouth: I feel it in my head

Collarbone: I don't know

Under Arm: That's okay

Top of Head: I'm a great kid

Eyebrow: It's okay if I don't know

Side of Eye: Sometimes I know right away

Under Eye: Sometimes it takes longer

Under Nose: And that's okay

Under Mouth: I'm a great kid!

Collarbone: I can do this!

Under Arm: I can let go of this feeling in my head

Top of Head: I can do this!

Eyebrow: I'm a great kid

Side of Eye: Everything's okay

Under Eye: I can figure it out

Under Nose: I'm an awesome kid

Under Mouth: And everything's okay!

Collarbone: I can do this!

Under Arm: This can feel easy for me!

Top of Head: I'm a great kid and I can do this!

If, like Gabrielle's son, your child is now willing to do whatever it is they felt they couldn't do, great! If they're still resistant, have them rate how true the belief feels now, and keep Tapping. For some kids, focusing more on physical sensations is especially powerful; others respond more to Tapping on releasing emotions.

Overcoming Anxiety Outbursts

Tom, 6 years old, was having trouble in class. He often got frustrated, and then so angry that his behavior would disrupt his classmates. At that point he had to be removed from the classroom. Every time that happened, he explained that his work wasn't "good enough," when in fact his work was often above average.

The teacher had hoped his issues would dissipate as the school year progressed, but instead, Tom's tantrums were becoming a bigger problem. More and more, his anger and frustration were preventing him from completing his assignments. His outbursts were also interfering with his classmates' ability to learn.

Knowing that his parents were getting a divorce and that his mother had been diagnosed with breast cancer, Tom's teacher wanted to give him a way to release his emotions that she hoped might allow him to feel safe when he made mistakes or did work that he didn't like.

To give Tom some positive protective distancing from his emotions, she used a puppet. The puppet, a silly cat named Meow, asked Tom some questions. Through talking to Meow, Tom realized that the issue isn't just about his work not being "good enough," it's also the anger he feels when that happens.

Before beginning to tap, Meow asked Tom how mad he feels when he does work that he feels isn't "good enough." Tom spread his arms wide open to show that he felt really mad when that happened. This is a powerful way of measuring emotional intensity with younger kids, who may sometimes find it hard to give their emotions a number on a scale of 0 to 10.

Meow then helped Tom create a setup statement that addressed both his feeling that his work isn't good enough and the anger that overtakes him when that happens. The setup statement was something like this:

"Even though my work is not good enough, my teacher wants me to finish it anyway. This makes me really mad, and I don't want to finish bad work…I'm still a good boy and I'm doing the best I can."

After Tapping through the points a few times, Tom seemed calmer. When asked how big his anger felt now, he brought his hands closer, indicating that his anger was much less intense.

Hoping to test his progress and see if his anger resurfaced when he did work that he felt wasn't "good enough," the teacher asked Tom to create a picture book of 3 things that he does well. She also lets him know that Meow can help him tap if he gets frustrated at any point in the project.

About 15 minutes into it, Tom became visibly agitated, frustrated by the drawing he was creating of himself playing soccer. Noticing this, the teacher suggested that he tap with Meow. Tom agreed and shared that he was feeling "this mad," opening his hands halfway. After Tapping through some rounds with Meow on his anger, Tom calmly completed his soccer picture and the entire picture book. At the end of the project, he seemed satisfied, and returned Meow to his home in the classroom.

As the year continued to progress, his teacher continued to give Tom access to Meow. As a result, most of the time Tom was able to complete his assignments and calm himself before his anger disrupted the class. Huge progress!

Your Takeaways…

Situations like this are powerful in a couple of ways:

- By giving Tom access to Meow and allowing him to tap when he's feeling frustrated and angry, the teacher was able to prevent his emotional outbursts from interfering with his learning.

- In addition, this early introduction to Tapping may plant a seed for Tom, giving him a way to manage his emotions as he gets older.

Child Tapping: Quieting Anxiety-Fueled Outbursts

When performance anxiety creates anger and tantrum-like behavior, begin by having your child rate his/her primary emotion—anger, frustration or other—on a scale of 0 to 10 or by using the "this much" method of measurement.

Then begin Tapping:

Karate Chop *(Repeat 3 times)*: Even though I'm so mad/frustrated/etc., I'm a great kid and I'm okay.

Eyebrow: So mad right now!

Side of Eye: So frustrated!

Under Eye: It's too hard

Under Nose: And I hate it

Under Mouth: I can't do it

Collarbone: So mad right now

Under Arm: That's okay

Top of Head: Still mad, though!

Eyebrow: I hate this

Side of Eye: That's okay

Under Eye: I'm a great kid!

Under Nose: I can do this!

Under Mouth: Everything's okay!

Collarbone: I can practice this

Under Arm: I can figure it out!

Top of Head: I'm a great kid and I can do this!

Have your child rate the intensity of his or her primary emotion again. Continue Tapping until s/he gets the desired relief.

Addressing Competition/Contest Anxiety

For some people competing is fun; for others, it's torture. This story is a great example of how Tapping can transform the experience of competing into a positive experience, even for those who initially dread it.

Mari began Tapping with her mom when she first began competing in scholar contests at 11 years old. A gifted child, Mari excelled academically, but suffered from performance anxiety as a result of the competitions. Thanks to Tapping, Mari was able to overcome her performance anxiety and excel at school and in competitions.

Now a teenager, Mari continues to use Tapping to quiet test anxiety, and also as a way to focus. As she has grown older, she's also successfully used Tapping to believe in herself and adjust to the many changes involved in growing up. Mari is thriving in every way and continues to use Tapping whenever she needs it.

I love this story, mostly because of how Tapping has helped Mari to develop a sense of self that extends beyond her academic achievements. By Tapping on her anxiety and other emotions over the years, she's been able to develop a broader and more solid sense of self. That solid foundation will serve her well throughout her life.

Let's look now at how to use Tapping as a tool to help your child prepare for whatever competition they may be involved in, from academics to sports, the arts and beyond.

Child Tapping: **Preparing for Competition**

Whether it's a spelling bee, theater audition, sports try-out or something else, if your child is anxious about competing or trying out, Tapping is a great way to calm their nerves, both as they prepare to compete and immediately before they engage in the competition.

Begin by having your child rate their performance anxiety, either on a scale of 0 to 10 or using the "this much" method of measurement.

Take a deep breath and begin Tapping.

Karate Chop *(Repeat 3 times)*: Even though I'm so anxious about this competition, and it's hard to even concentrate, I'm okay.

Eyebrow: This competition...

Side of Eye: Making me so nervous

Under Eye: So anxious

Under Nose: I can feel it in my body

Under Mouth: This competition

Collarbone: Making me feel so anxious!

Under Arm: I can feel it in my body

Top of Head: It's hard to focus when I feel so nervous

Eyebrow: All this nervousness

Side of Eye: So much anxiety about this competition

Under Eye: It's okay to feel this

Under Nose: I really want to do my best

Under Mouth: But I'm scared I won't

Collarbone: What if I mess up?

Under Arm: What if I don't mess up?

Top of Head: Maybe I'll do really well!

Eyebrow: I can focus on preparing

Side of Eye: It's safe to let go of this anxiety

Under Eye: And feel relaxed and calm in my body

Under Nose: I can do this!

Under Mouth: I'll do my best!

Collarbone: That's what matters

Under Arm: Letting go of this anxiety now

Top of Head: Feeling relaxed and confident

Have your child rate their performance anxiety once again, and keep Tapping until they get the desired relief.

Getting Ready To Step On Stage

This story is from Kathryn, whose niece had begun performing in dance recitals at a young age.

During her niece's first time on stage, she'd been so afraid that a teacher had to carry her around on stage during the performance.

Hoping to help her overcome her intense stage fright, the following year, Kathryn made sure to do Tapping with her, both during rehearsals in the weeks before the performance and immediately before stepping on stage.

To Kathryn's delight and amazement, her niece transformed into a confident performer, dancing her part beautifully and enjoying every minute she spent on stage.

We've all heard stories like this, and without thinking twice, downplayed their significance. *Oh, that's nice*, we think. *That little girl did well in her dance recital.* After years of helping people work through their fears and phobias, though, I've seen again and again how profoundly one negative experience can limit us. Getting laughed at once, forgetting your lines once, or tripping on stage once is often all it takes to create stage fright that lasts a lifetime. By using Tapping to overcome her stage fright so early, Kathryn's niece is now free of her fears, and ready to thrive both on stage and off. That's huge!

Let's take a look next at how to use Tapping immediately before a performance or competition.

Child Tapping: **Stepping Out on Stage (or on the Field, etc.)**

On the day of the big show, game or performance, it's great to tap once (or several times!), first focusing on calming anxiety and then while visualizing success.

To begin doing that, first have your child rate their performance anxiety, either on a scale of 0 to 10 or using the "this much" method of measurement.

Take a deep breath and begin Tapping.

Karate Chop *(Repeat 3 times)*: Even though I feel so anxious about this performance, because it's the big day and I'm scared, I'm a great kid and I'm okay.

Eyebrow: Ahh, it's the big day!

Side of Eye: So nervous!

Under Eye: So much anxiety

Under Nose: I feel it in my body

Under Mouth: I really want to do well

Collarbone: But I'm scared

Under Arm: So nervous!

Top of Head: So scared!

Eyebrow: That's okay

Side of Eye: It's normal to feel this way

Under Eye: I can let myself feel it all now

Under Nose: And I can let it all go

Under Mouth: I can do this!

Collarbone: I'm a great kid no matter what

Under Arm: I can relax now

Top of Head: I can feel safe now

Eyebrow: I can do this!

Side of Eye: I can relax and focus on what I need to do

Under Eye: I can feel safe and calm in my body

Under Nose: It's safe to feel calm now

Under Mouth: It's safe to feel excited about performing

Collarbone: I don't have to worry

Under Arm: I'm a great kid no matter what

Top of Head: I can do this!

Have your child rate his or her performance anxiety again, and keep Tapping until s/he gets the desired relief.

When your child is ready, have him/her continue Tapping through the points while visualizing a successful outcome. S/he doesn't have to describe what that outcome is, just have her/him visualize what success looks like in his/her mind (or out loud, if s/he prefers).

Encourage your child to feel what success will feel like. Keep Tapping through a few rounds until s/he can visualize that success with minimal anxiety or nervousness.

Remind your child also that s/he can tap in the bathroom, locker room, or in the wings of the stage—and of course, if s/he is willing, a big hug never hurts!

TAPPING WITH YOUR CHILD: SCHOOL JITTERS

New classmates, new teachers, new classroom, new material to learn—there's not much about the start of a school year that *isn't* new. Not surprisingly, kids often get first-day-of-school jitters. As we'll see in this section, Tapping is a powerful way to reduce the anxiety many kids experience before their first day of school, as well as the first day of camp and other important "first" days.

Since you may also worry about how they'll do or feel on this very important day, we'll begin by doing some Tapping to reduce your stress. Once you've had an experience, we'll then look at how to use Tapping with your child.

Adult Tapping: Releasing the Stress of Your Child's School Jitters

How much stress or anxiety do you feel when you think about your child's first day of school? Do you feel worried about how s/he will perform academically, whether s/he will make friends, pay attention to the teacher, or succeed in extracurricular activities?

If not, imagine yourself starting a new job or joining a new organization that required that you perform in some way.

Rate your stress and anxiety on a scale of 0 to 10.

Take a deep breath. Let's begin by Tapping 3 times on the Karate Chop point:

Karate Chop (*Repeat 3 times*): Even though I feel anxious about this situation that seems out of my control, I deeply and completely love and accept myself.

Eyebrow: All this anxiety

Side of Eye: So much anxiety

Under Eye: Not sure how this will turn out

Under Nose: Not sure about the outcome

Under Mouth: Wish I could make sure it worked out

Collarbone: Wish I could make my child feel comfortable about this

Under Arm: Wish I could take away their anxiety

Top of Head: Letting myself feel my anxiety now

Eyebrow: I feel powerless to fix this

Side of Eye: I wish I could help her feel excited

Under Eye: I'm anxious about this, too

Under Nose: Letting myself feel this anxiety now

Under Mouth: And letting it all go

Collarbone: Letting myself fully feel my anxiety now

Under Arm: And releasing it now

Top of Head: Even though I can't change the situation

Eyebrow: I can let go of this anxiety now

Side of Eye: Releasing any remaining stress and anxiety now

Under Eye: Allowing myself to trust that everything will be fine

Under Nose: Relaxing when I think about this unknown situation

Under Mouth: Letting go of any leftover stress and anxiety

Collarbone: Allowing myself to relax and feel calm now

Under Arm: I can trust that this will work out

Top of Head: Allowing myself to feel relaxed and calm now

Take another deep breath, and rate your stress and anxiety once again. Keep Tapping until you get the desired relief.

Next, let's look at how to tap with your child on how s/he can release first-day-of-school jitters.

Note: As always, when Tapping with your child, tailor your words to your child's age and experience.

First Day of "Big Kid" School

Yet another active summer had flown by, and now there was just one week left before my 6-year-old nephew, Malakai, would be starting 1st grade at a new school. He had loved the school he'd attended for the past 3 years. Throughout that time, he'd been in the same classroom with the same teacher, and had thrived—he'd even assumed a leadership role toward the younger kids.

Knowing how driven Malakai is by certainty, Karen and Alex, his parents, wondered how he'd been feeling about his upcoming school transition. His behavior had been erratic all summer, but he hadn't been interested in talking about his new school. When they'd asked if he wanted to tap, he usually said no. Wanting to respect his boundaries and feelings, they hadn't forced him to discuss it.

With summer quickly coming to a close, however, it seemed important to address the topic. While putting Malakai to bed one night, Karen asked him how he was feeling about going to a new school. Looking a bit anxious, he immediately snuggled into her. She asked him gently if he'd like to tap, and this time he said yes.

Karen then tapped through the points on him, while he, in turn, tapped through the points on her. It was a very sweet moment.

As they tapped on each other, Karen began describing all of the concerns she imagined he might have—about what his new teacher might be like, what his classroom would look like, whether he'd make friends, what he would need to do to ride the school bus, and more. When they finished Tapping, Malakai's energy shifted completely. Rather than seeming anxious, he was visibly excited, asking questions about his new school, the school bus and more.

The following day, they all attended an orientation at his new school. After hearing the school principal speak, they visited Malakai's new classroom. To make him feel comfortable in his new surroundings, Karen walked him around the room, pointing out where the kids would create art, sit for circle and so forth. They noticed where his school supplies were kept, and he was able to find his desk, as well.

By his first day of school, Malakai's excitement had grown exponentially. He came home from school excited and energized, reporting that he'd gotten to play on the monkey bars at the new school, which had been his favorite part of recess in kindergarten at his old school. He quickly made friends, bonded with his teacher and was soon thriving as a happy first-grader in his new school!

Child Tapping: Overcoming "Big Kid School" Jitters

Have your child rate his or her "icky" or nervous feeling about the first day at a new, bigger school using a 0 to 10 scale or the "this much" method of measurement.

Then begin by Tapping 3 times on the Karate Chop point:

Karate Chop (*Repeat 3 times*): Even though I'm so nervous about my first day of "big kid" school, I'm an awesome kid and I'm okay.

Eyebrow: I don't know what it's going to be like

Side of Eye: I don't even know my teacher

Under Eye: Will I make new friends?

Under Nose: What will the school bus be like?

Under Mouth: I don't know what it'll be like

Collarbone: Who will I play with?

Under Arm: What's my teacher like?

Top of Head: Will I like my new school?

Eyebrow: Where will my classroom be?

Side of Eye: Will I make new friends?

Under Eye: I'm so nervous!

Under Nose: Everything will be new

Under Mouth: Maybe it'll be really exciting

Collarbone: Maybe I'll love my new school

Under Arm: I'll probably make lots of new friends

Top of Head: It could be really fun!

Eyebrow: It's okay that everything will be new

Side of Eye: I'm a great kid!

Under Eye: And I'm okay!

Under Nose: I can feel calm about my new school

Under Mouth: Even though it's all new

Collarbone: I can feel calm when I think about it

Under Arm: It might be really fun!

Top of Head: I'm a great kid and I'm okay!

Ask your child to rate his or her jitters once again. As always, keep Tapping until s/he gets the desired relief.

The New School Bus Rider

When a new school year means that your child will be riding the school bus for the first time, that school bus routine can be an extra cause of stress.

For Alex and Karen, that issue came to light during an open house at Malakai's new elementary school. (What can I say…? I'm writing a book about families…I figured I *had to* include some stories about my own!)

While talking to his teacher, Alex and Karen learned that Malakai had been very serious in school. That wasn't a huge surprise, since he tended to be serious

In new situations. The teacher then mentioned that Malakai seemed to be very anxious about missing the school bus at the end of the day.

That evening when they returned home, after telling Malakai how proud of him they were, Alex brought up the topic of the bus at the end of the school day. Malakai nodded, and shared that he gets nervous about missing it. The way it works, he explained, is that the kids need to go outside when their bus number is called. Often, though, friends are talking and playing and it's hard to hear which number is being called. Every day he worries that he'll miss his bus.

Alex asked him if he'd like to tap on it, and he said yes.

They did some Tapping together, with Alex Tapping on him as Malakai repeated the phrases that Alex said. Using statements like, "Even though I get nervous about missing the bus, I love and accept myself," and "Even though I get nervous about not hearing my bus number and missing the bus, I love and accept myself, and I know I'm a good kid." They tapped together for a few minutes.

After doing some rounds on the "negatives"—Malakai's nervousness, fears of missing his bus, etc.—they then moved on to positive statements like, "Even if I miss the bus, I know everything will be okay."

Once they had transitioned to the positive rounds, Malakai's energy shifted. He suddenly blurted out, "Yeah, and if I miss the bus, you or mummy are allowed to come pick me up at the school." Alex nodded, and together they continued Tapping on the positive. He then felt tired, and said he wanted to go to bed. Alex asked him if he felt better about the bus, and he said that he did.

He then asked Alex if he would speak in the voice of "Henry" (his stuffed dinosaur, who had long ago been given an English accent), and Alex did. Together, they did some Tapping on Henry around missing Malakai when he's not home. Malakai did the Tapping on Henry.

By the end of their Tapping, both Henry and Malakai went to bed feeling happy and relaxed.

Since Tapping on releasing his fear, Malakai has been able to relax about his daily bus rides, knowing that mom or dad will come and pick him up if he ever misses the bus. That's a huge improvement in how safe he feels being out in the world. That basic sense of safety will likely serve him well in the years to come, creating a solid foundation for healthy, positive self-esteem.

Child Tapping: Feeling at Ease Riding the School Bus

First ask your child how s/he feels about riding the school bus. Have her or him rate her or his feelings on a scale of 0 to 10 or using the "this much" method of measurement.

Let's begin by Tapping 3 times on the Karate Chop point:

Karate Chop *(Repeat 3 times)*: Even though I feel a little yucky about the school bus, I'm a great kid and I'm okay.

Eyebrow: Not sure about riding the school bus

Side of Eye: It looks kind of fun

Under Eye: But I'm really not sure

Under Nose: I don't even get how it works!

Under Mouth: What if I miss it?

Collarbone: What if I miss my stop?

Under Arm: All this icky feeling about the school bus

Top of Head: So many big kids

Eyebrow: Not sure about it

Side of Eye: What if they're mean to me?

Under Eye: Maybe it could be fun

Under Nose: Maybe I'll like it

Under Mouth: I can ask for help if I need it

Collarbone: I'm okay

Under Arm: I can let go of this icky feeling

Top of Head: And ask for help when I need it

Eyebrow: I'm a great kid!

Side of Eye: And I'm okay

Under Eye: Letting go of this icky feeling about the bus

Under Nose: I can feel calmer when I think about the school bus

Under Mouth: I'm a great kid

Collarbone: And I'm okay

Under Arm: I can feel calm when I think about the school bus

Top of Head: I'm a great kid and I'm okay!

Ask your child to rate his or her "icky" (or nervous, etc.) feeling about the school bus now. Keep Tapping until s/he gets the desired relief.

Easing the Transition to a New School Year

Even after the first day has come and gone, kids may struggle with the many transitions inherent in the start of a new school year for days, if not weeks, afterward. That was the case for Alexandra, who, at bedtime after the second day of a new school year, was having trouble settling down for her bedtime story.

When she finally sat down on her bed, she burst into tears. She explained to her mom and dad that she was nervous about school. She'd been having difficulty finishing her in-class assignments, and hadn't yet made any friends. It was all really overwhelming, and she didn't want to go back.

They all began Tapping together, and continued to include Tapping in their nightly bedtime ritual. By the end of that week, Alexandra was coming home from school talking about her new friends, and also about how much easier it had been to complete her work. Just those few minutes of Tapping before bed each night had completely changed her school experience!

Child Tapping: Overcoming New School Year Nervousness

The best way to start Tapping on your child's challenges around a new school year is first to talk with him or her about what's happening. Is s/he struggling socially, academically or both? How does s/he feel about her or his new teacher, classroom, schedule and so on? If it helps to tap while s/he talks, then do that. If s/he prefers to share first, that's fine, too.

Once you're clearer on the challenges s/he is struggling with, have her or him rate how hard it feels on a scale of 0 to 10 or using the "this much" method of measurement.

Then begin by Tapping 3 times on the Karate Chop point:

Karate Chop *(Repeat 3 times)*: Even though I'm feeling so nervous about this new part of school, I'm an awesome kid and I'm okay.

Eyebrow: Feeling really icky

Side of Eye: Not sure how I feel about school this year

Under Eye: Everything's so new

Under Nose: It doesn't feel good

Under Mouth: Feeling yucky/nervous about school

Collarbone: It's all so new

Under Arm: I'm not sure I like it

Top of Head: Feeling yucky about school this year

Eyebrow: That's okay

Side of Eye: It's all so new

Under Eye: And I'm a great kid

Under Nose: And I'm okay

Under Mouth: Still not sure how I feel about school this year

Collarbone: But I'm a great kid

Under Arm: And I'm okay

Top of Head: I can feel calm about school now

Eyebrow: Even though everything's so new

Side of Eye: I'm still a great kid

Under Eye: And I'm okay

Under Nose: I can feel calm when I think about school

Under Mouth: I'm okay

Collarbone: I'm a great kid!

Under Arm: And I'm okay

Top of Head: I can feel calm now when I think about school

Ask your child to rate his or her feeling about school now. Keep Tapping until s/he gets the desired relief.

First Day of High School

Few things are more overwhelming and intimidating to teenagers than walking into a building filled mostly with kids who are older, bigger, and faster—kids who know more and can do more than they can. That can be how many kids feel when they're first starting high school.

For Betty's son, Nolan, the jitters hit the night before the first day of his freshman year of high school. He felt nervous, sure that he wasn't yet ready. His anxiety grew so intense at bedtime, in fact, that he couldn't fall asleep. When he confessed his anxiety to his mom, she tapped with him for a half hour. They went through everything he was nervous about—from not being able to keep up academically to anxiety about fitting in socially, worry about trying out for sports and other extracurricular activities, and more. When they were finished Tapping, he fell asleep and slept through the night. The next morning, his first-day-of-school nerves were completely gone, and he went on to have a great first day of high school.

Child/Teenager Tapping: Overcoming First-Day-of-High-School (or Middle School) Jitters

First ask your child if s/he is especially nervous about any one or two things—the social scene, academics, sports try-outs, etc. If it helps to tap as s/he talks, do that. If not, listen as s/he shares what's on her or his mind.

When s/he is ready to begin Tapping, ask your child how nervous or anxious s/he feels about those issues on a scale of 0 to 10.

Take a deep breath together, and then begin by Tapping 3 times on the Karate Chop point. This script will touch on several topics, but if your child is primarily focused on one or two, focus your Tapping on what s/he is feeling.

Karate Chop *(Repeat 3 times)*: Even though I'm really nervous about starting this new school and I don't know if I'm ready for it, I'm cool and it's okay.

Eyebrow: Not sure I'm ready

Side of Eye: I feel really nervous

Under Eye: I don't feel ready

Under Nose: I'm scared I won't make friends

Under Mouth: I'm worried about my classes

Collarbone: And all those new teachers

Under Arm: I don't feel ready for this new school

Top of Head: I'm so anxious

Eyebrow: It's okay to feel this way

Side of Eye: It's all new

Under Eye: And that's okay

Under Nose: It's okay to feel nervous

Under Mouth: I can handle this!

Collarbone: I'm a great girl/guy

Under Arm: Everything will be new

Top of Head: It might feel weird at first

Eyebrow: That's okay

Side of Eye: I can take it one day at a time

Under Eye: I don't have to worry

Under Nose: I can relax about it

Under Mouth: And take the changes one at a time

Collarbone: I'm okay

Under Arm: I can relax about my new school

Top of Head: I'm okay, and I can relax now

Have your child rate his or her anxiety about the new school now. Keep Tapping until s/he gets the desired relief.

TAPPING WITH YOUR CHILD: BULLYING

While our growing awareness around bullying is an important step forward, bullying continues to be a daily reality for far too many kids. Using Tapping, we can move beyond awareness and help kids who have been bullied to regain their self-esteem and shed the shame they may feel. We can also help bullies, many of whom were bullied themselves and may also be dealing with trauma, to heal their own wounds.

Before we look at how to use Tapping, let's step back and look at what bullying is. According to StopBullying.gov, a government website managed by the U.S. Department of Health & Human Services[1], bullying is defined as:

- Unwanted, aggressive behavior among school-aged children that involves a real or perceived power imbalance. The behavior is repeated, or has the potential to be repeated, over time. Both kids who are bullied and who bully others may have serious, lasting problems.

In order to be considered bullying, the behavior must be aggressive and include:

- An Imbalance of Power: Kids who bully use their power—such as physical strength, access to embarrassing information, or popularity—to control or harm others. Power imbalances can change over time and in different situations, even if they involve the same people.

- Repetition: Bullying behaviors happen more than once or have the potential to happen more than once.

Bullying includes actions such as making threats, spreading rumors, attacking someone physically or verbally, and excluding someone from a group on purpose.

The effects of bullying can be intense and overwhelming, both for kids and their parents, who often feel helpless to stop bullying that happens at school or elsewhere when they're not present to interfere.

Before we begin Tapping with your child, let's first shed some of your stress around this issue.

Adult Tapping: Releasing Angst over Bullying

When you think about your child being bullied, what emotion do you feel most intensely—fear, anger, or other? Focus on the emotion that feels most intense at this moment, and give it a number of intensity on a scale of 0 to 10.

In this Tapping script, I'll focus on fear and anger, but as always, use words that reflect your experience.

To begin, take a deep breath, and let's start by Tapping 3 times on the Karate Chop point.

Karate Chop *(Repeat 3 times)*: Even though I'm so angry and afraid about my child being bullied, I deeply and completely love and accept myself.

Eyebrow: So much fear

Side of Eye: So much anger

Under Eye: I'm terrified what this is doing to her

Under Nose: I'm terrified I'm not doing enough

Under Mouth: I'm so angry that this is happening

Collarbone: I'm so angry at the kids who are doing the bullying

Under Arm: I'm so angry!

Top of Head: And so scared

Eyebrow: What will this do to her confidence?

Side of Eye: I feel so powerless

Under Eye: I'm so scared about what bullying is doing to my child

Under Nose: I feel so powerless to help him

Under Mouth: So much fear

Collarbone: So much anger

Under Arm: Letting myself feel it now

Top of Head: And letting it go

Eyebrow: Releasing it from every cell in my body now

Side of Eye: I'm not powerless

Under Eye: This is so hard

Under Nose: But we're going to work through this

Under Mouth: Letting go of this fear and anger now

Collarbone: I can let go of this fear and anger

Under Arm: And feel hopeful and safe

Top of Head: And empowered to transform this situation

Take a deep breath, and check back in on the fear and anger, or other emotion. Give them a number on a scale of 0 to 10. Keep Tapping until you feel more grounded and ready to be present with your child.

Note: As always, when Tapping with your child, tailor your words to your child's age and experience.

Releasing Memories of Being Bullied

Even when bullying has long since passed, it can have a lasting impact on a child's daily experience. This story shows how Tapping can help kids to release the emotional residue created by bullying, even when that bullying happened years beforehand.

Sarah was in 2nd grade when she began having a panic attack at bedtime one night. Concerned, her mom, Jean, asked if she could tap through the points while Sarah shared what was going on. Sarah nodded yes. As her mom tapped through the points on Sarah's body, Sarah shared that her anxiety had started when she'd thought about a time on the school bus during her first week of kindergarten.

Although 3 years had gone by since then, her memory still felt very real. That day, she'd been so excited to be on the "big kids" bus. Soon after sitting down, though, other kids on the bus had turned to her and told her they were going to kill her. They also began singing a song about Sarah's mom, saying she had a "really huge, big butt."

Recalling the memory 3 years later, Sarah shared that she wished she could hurt those kids the way they'd hurt her. Her mom kept Tapping through the points as Sarah continued to tell the story. More than their threat to kill her, it was the insults toward her mom that had made Sarah so mad. As Sarah's mood lightened and her body relaxed, her mom made a joke about her own butt. They both giggled, and Sarah promptly fell asleep.

A few months later, they were riding in the car when Sir Mix-a-Lot's song "Baby Got Back" came on the radio. Without realizing it, Jean began singing along. Sarah immediately asked, "How do you know that song?" Jean explained that it was a popular song from years ago, so lots of people know it. "Oh," Sarah replied. "That was the song those kids were singing about you on the bus." Jean smiled and started singing even louder. They both collapsed into a big, long belly laugh.

Child Tapping: **Moving beyond Bullying**

If your child is being bullied, ask if s/he is willing to tap through the points while talking about what's happening.

Since bullying is a painful topic for many kids, do your best to be fully present and tap along with him or her as s/he speaks.

Instead of offering to help (by contacting the school, etc.), or even labeling anyone as a "bully," give your child your full presence by listening as s/he voices her or his experiences and emotions.

Let him/her continue to tap and talk until the emotional charge is significantly lower. Once s/he is feeling safer and more relaxed, s/he may be more open to talking about any action steps or behavioral changes that may protect her/him from further bullying.

"I Hate School!"

Since children don't always share the details of their experience, it's not always clear when bullying is the root cause of behavioral changes and patterns. This story shows how Tapping can be used both as a discovery tool and an emotional processing/healing tool.

The school year was about to begin, and Scott, 7 years old, was protesting, saying that he hated school. Unable to change his mind about school, his mother called in an EFT practitioner, whom they called "the coach," to help Scott adjust to the new school year.

After completing the first round of Tapping with Scott, "the coach" asked Scott what was bothering him. Without hesitation, he replied, "I am angry about having to go to school." Scott then explained that another boy in his class, Nathan, had been picking on him since kindergarten.

Together, Scott and "the coach" began Tapping, using the setup statement, "Even though I am so angry about being bullied by Nathan, I deeply and completely accept myself." After Tapping through his first round, Scott began to cry, and shared that it felt so good to talk about this. He also said that his body felt looser as he tapped. That was unusual, he added, since his body usually tensed up when he thought about Nathan. However, he still didn't want anyone to know that Nathan was singling him out at school.

With more Tapping, Scott's anger decreased significantly. That seemed to be a relief, but Kyle shared that he had another problem. While he didn't feel as angry, he was still afraid of Nathan. He didn't know how to handle Nathan's teasing or the "evil eye" he frequently gave Scott, which made Scott think Nathan might beat him up. Whenever they were at school, Scott shared, he felt like Nathan was always nearby, waiting to "get me."

After doing more Tapping, Scott was able to relax again. After several rounds of Tapping, "the coach" asked him how he felt now about telling his mother about Nathan. Scott said that would be okay. Up until that point, Scott had never told his mother about how Nathan had been treating him.

Hoping to continue easing Scott's transition into school, she asked "the coach" to work with him more. They met twice per week for the following month. During that time, Scott also began Tapping every day. As a result, he was able to release all of his anger at Nathan. His entire attitude about school also changed, becoming more positive than it had ever been before. His confidence increased noticeably, as well.

3 months later, at Scott's mother's request, "the coach" returned to check in with Scott. When "the coach" asked Scott if he was still angry about being bullied, Scott looked surprised and then laughed. The intense anger and fear he'd felt had gone away completely. His mother has since shared that Scott is doing really well in school.

Reading this story, one of the first things that came to mind is how important it was to address Scott's experiences and emotions at such a young age. Giving him that opportunity to release his anger and fear at just 7 years old probably changed his life. It gave him the chance to feel safe at school, and as a result, he could then fully engage in learning. Without that opportunity to tap through his emotions and experiences, he understandably might have hated school forever.

Over time Scott might have resorted to bullying other kids in order to protect himself from being bullied again. That's an important point that we, as parents, need to keep in mind. Kids like Nathan often become bullies after being bullied themselves. They may also resort to bullying behavior as a result of being abused, or because of painful circumstances at home or elsewhere in their lives.

While it's understandable that we'd want to label and blame a child who is hurting our own, it's also important to consider that the child we're labeling as a "bully" may be in equal, if not greater, pain. If we, as adults, can do our own Tapping on how we feel about our child being bullied, we'll be better able to help our children not only to feel confident, loved and lovable, but also to grow into positive, compassionate adults. In other words, when we can feel compassion for others, we can teach it to our children.

Child Tapping: **Releasing Anger and Fear from Being Bullied**

Understandably, when a child becomes a target for bullying, s/he often experiences a range of emotions, including intense anger and fear, as well as a keen sense of powerlessness and the inability to change the situation. If your child isn't able or willing to share more about what's going on, you can also tap with her/him on the emotions s/he is feeling.

Begin first by measuring the intensity of those emotions, either on a scale of 0 to 10 or using the "this much" method of measurement.

Take a deep breath and then begin by Tapping 3 times on the Karate Chop point:

Karate Chop *(Repeat 3 times)*: Even though I'm so mad and scared about what they're doing to me, I'm a great kid and I'm okay.

Eyebrow: So mad!

Side of Eye: So mad at how they treat me

Under Eye: It's scary

Under Nose: I freeze when it happens

Under Mouth: It's so scary

Collarbone: I can't respond

Under Arm: I freeze when it happens

Top of Head: It's so scary

Eyebrow: And it also makes me so mad

Side of Eye: I want to hurt them!

Under Eye: They make me feel bad

Under Nose: It makes me feel so bad

Under Mouth: But I'm a great kid

Collarbone: And it's not my fault

Under Arm: They're making bad choices

Top of Head: But I'm a great kid

Eyebrow: I don't like how it makes me feel

Side of Eye: It makes me mad and sad

Under Eye: It makes me feel sad

Under Nose: But I'm a great kid!

Under Mouth: They're making bad choices

Collarbone: But I'm a great kid

Under Arm: And I'm okay!

Top of Head: I'm a great kid, and everything's okay

Ask your child to take a deep breath and rate his/her emotions—anger, fear, sadness, and whatever else s/he feels about being bullied—again. Keep Tapping until s/he gets the desired relief.

From Bully to Enlightened Leader

Bullies are made, not born, and yet many of us struggle to feel compassion for them. This is completely understandable—they are hurting our children! But what then happens is that bullies lose their voice, often even their right to speak—except when they're behaving like bullies, and so the cycle perpetuates itself.

So what happens when we go out of our way to give bullies a voice—and then a chance to heal from the pain that is causing them to behave like bullies? It was the question The Tapping Solution Foundation got an opportunity to answer when we first began working with Shyla.

During her last year in middle school, Shyla had suddenly turned into a dark, brooding teenager. Now in high school, her grades had been in a downward spiral, and nearly every week she was being sent to the principal's office for bullying. Prone to rage-fueled outbursts, Shyla had become a source of disruption and frustration for teachers and administrators alike. Unfortunately, the ongoing negative attention she was getting—in the form of school detention, reprimands, and more—only seemed to worsen her attitude, behavior and performance.

What few at her school initially realized was that Shyla's transformation had taken place soon after a shooting occurred at her former school. Forced to remain still and quiet in the dark for five agonizingly long hours of citywide lockdown, Shyla, then a middle schooler, had huddled alone under a desk, listening for gunshots while helicopters flew overhead and sirens blared nearby. Although she had survived that day, all these years later Shyla was being haunted by the trauma of that experience. To make matters worse, Shyla's family life was unpredictable. Whether at home or school, Shyla felt she had nowhere to turn for support and guidance.

Fortunately, one administrator at her current school looked into Shyla's history. After realizing that Shyla had been caught in that shooting, the school reached out to The Tapping Solution Foundation, which is increasingly being recognized nationwide for the success of its trauma relief programs in schools.

Soon after sitting down with Shyla, it was clear to Dr. Lori Leyden of The Tapping Solution Foundation that Shyla was suffering from untreated Post-Traumatic Stress Disorder (PTSD) incurred during the school shooting. After explaining how Tapping accesses the amygdala in the brain and then lowers cortisol levels in the body, Dr. Leyden asked how her body feels when she's overcome by rage. Shyla described a burning sensation in her stomach and an inability to think before acting out her rage.

Hoping to motivate her to do trauma-healing work, Dr. Leyden asked Shyla what her goal was. Kids who are labeled as "bullies" are often punished, but rarely asked what they want or how they feel, so giving Shyla a voice in the process was critical. "I want to improve my grades so I can transfer to the school I want to go to," Shyla replied without hesitation. While many of her teachers saw Shyla as an out-of-control problem student, it was clear that Shyla had done extensive independent research about attending this one specific school. In order to attend that school, however, she had to maintain a higher grade point average and receive positive reviews from teachers.

With that long-term goal clearly in mind, Dr. Leyden then asked Shyla to focus on a petty annoyance she'd recently experienced. Before diving into trauma healing work, it's important to experience some kind of results from Tapping, as those initial results allow people to become more invested in the process.

Shyla's petty annoyance had happened a few days earlier, when her sister had borrowed her favorite shirt without asking. Using that event as a starting point, Dr. Leyden led Shyla through a few rounds of Tapping. Within just a few minutes, Shyla could recall the event without feeling any irritation. She also shared that her body felt more relaxed.

Over a period of several weeks, Dr. Leyden conducted weekly Tapping sessions with Shyla, focusing on clearing the emotional intensity of her memories of the school shooting. When the focus turned to Shyla's bullying behavior, it became clear that she, like many kids, had only begun bullying others after being continually bullied by a small group of students at her current school. Her bullying was a coping strategy, a way to appear tough so that she herself would no longer be harassed.

There had been one especially traumatic day when a student had called her fat, and then ripped her shirt and pushed her into a nearby crowd to be publicly mocked. Just recalling that day, Shyla could feel rage burning in her stomach before racing up into her head. With that memory fresh in her mind, it took just two rounds of Tapping to get Shyla's rage from a 10 out of 10 down to a 2.

After releasing the emotional charge from these events and others, Shyla once again became a different kid. This time, however, the transformation was a reflection of her positive mental and emotional well-being. The next time she was bullied, instead of lashing out in rage, she stayed calm. She also reported the bullying to school administrators. Her goal of getting into that other school was so important to her that for the first time ever, Shyla was willing to risk being called a "tattletale."

Once she'd used Tapping to heal from the trauma of the school shooting that she'd experienced, Shyla no longer needed to use bullying behavior to defend herself. Instead, she can now rely on positive forms of leadership to move her life and school community forward. Shyla has become a leader at her school. Teachers and administrators alike now see her as an example of the transformation they want to see in other students.

Child Tapping: No Longer the Bully

If your child is acting out his/her emotions by bullying other children, it's likely a way of managing emotional pain that s/he is trying to handle. Rather than accusing or labeling your child, ask her/him how s/he feels when s/he teases, taunts, mocks or exhibits other negative behaviors.

As one example, if your child says that s/he feels angry when s/he acts that way, ask her/him to rate the intensity of that anger, either on a 0 to 10 scale or using the "this much" method of measurement.

Then lead her/him through Tapping, using statements like:

Karate Chop *(Repeat 3 times)*: Even though I have all this anger in my body, I'm a great kid and I'm okay.

Eyebrow: So much anger in my body

Side of Eye: It feels so big

Under Eye: All this anger in my body

Under Nose: So much anger in me

Under Mouth: I don't know what to do with it

Collarbone: I get so angry sometimes

Under Arm: All this anger in my body

Top of Head: I don't know what to do with it

Eyebrow: I get so angry sometimes

Side of Eye: I can feel it in my body

Under Eye: I don't know what to do with it

Under Nose: But I'm a great kid

Under Mouth: I feel bad sometimes

Collarbone: I get so mad sometimes

Under Arm: But I'm still a great kid

Top of Head: And I'm okay

Eyebrow: Letting myself feel this anger now

Side of Eye: Letting myself feel the anger in my body

Under Eye: And now I can let it go

Under Nose: I can let go of this anger now

Under Mouth: I'm a great kid

Collarbone: And I'm okay

Under Arm: I can use Tapping when I feel angry

Top of Head: I'm a great kid and I'm okay

Take a deep breath and ask your child to rate her/his anger one more time. Keep Tapping until s/he gets the desired relief.

Keeping in mind that most bullies have been bullied themselves. If your child is willing, you can then ask open-ended, non-judgmental questions like:

- Why do you get angry?
- Has anyone ever bullied you or treated you badly?

If s/he is willing to share, have her/him tap through the points as s/he tells the story. Continue Tapping until s/he can tell and retell the story without experiencing any emotional charge.

Whenever possible, try to establish a regular routine of Tapping on releasing emotions, processing social situations and letting go of any confusing or disturbing events or interactions that may have happened at school or elsewhere.

Chapter 13

Managing Challenging Relationships

TAPPING WITH YOUR CHILD: ADULTS

Navigating different types of relationships is often challenging for children. Whether those challenges arise with a parent, coach or teacher, Tapping can help your child to gain clarity on why certain relationship(s) challenge them, and how to change his/her experience within that relationship.

Since it's not possible to control how others act or react, the most powerful tool each of us can bring to relationships is an evolving awareness of our own selves—namely, how we feel and what we believe about people, relationships and ourselves.

Developing relationship skills is a lifelong process. We'll begin using Tapping in this section to better understand why certain relationships may feel especially challenging.

As always, the best place to begin is by releasing your own stress. We'll do that by Tapping on releasing any emotions you may feel when your relationship with your child feels strained.

Adult Tapping: **Releasing Stress Around Your Child's Resistance toward You**

How do you feel when your child is angry with you? When s/he shouts, "I hate you!" and runs away? What do you tell yourself when your child refuses to talk to you?

For this exercise focus on a specific instance or period of time when your relationship with your child was strained. How does that make you feel—fearful, anxious, ashamed, angry, sad…? Notice which emotion feels most intense and give it a number of intensity on a scale of 0 to 10.

As always, tailor your Tapping to your experience.

Begin by taking a deep breath and then Tapping 3 times on the Karate Chop point.

Karate Chop *(Repeat 3 times)*: Even though I feel all this stress around my child's relationship challenges with me, I deeply and completely love and accept myself.

Eyebrow: So stressful

Side of Eye: I'm trying so hard

Under Eye: And I feel like the enemy

Under Nose: This stress

Under Mouth: It's affecting our entire home and family life

Collarbone: I don't like feeling like this

Under Arm: All this stress

Top of Head: I don't know if I can fix it

Eyebrow: This stress

Side of Eye: It's overwhelming

Under Eye: It's frustrating

Under Nose: It's okay to let myself feel it now

Under Mouth: And to let it go

Collarbone: It's safe to feel this stress now

Under Arm: And it's safe to let it go

Top of Head: I don't love how hard my relationship with my child feels right now

Eyebrow: But it's still safe to let go of my stress around it

Side of Eye: I can give him/her the space s/he needs

Under Eye: And feel safe letting go of this stress now

Under Nose: I can trust that this will pass

Under Mouth: I can trust in my own parenting instincts

Collarbone: Even though it's not always easy

Under Arm: I can let go of this stress now

Top of Head: And let myself relax when I think about our relationship challenges

Take a deep breath, and notice how intensely you feel your primary emotion(s) now. Keep Tapping until you get the relief you desire.

Getting to Core Relationship Issues

Developing healthy relationship skills starts with learning to ask the right types of questions. Those questions lead to increased self-awareness, which supports healthier relationships.

For example, if your child is struggling due to a coach who is pushing him/her to perform at a higher level, first let your child vent his/her feelings without judging or commenting on what s/he is sharing.

Next, as you both tap through the points, ask your child questions like:

- How do you feel when you think about this person?
- Is there an event or remark that comes to mind when you think of this person?

- How do you feel about yourself when you're with this person?

Your child's answers to these questions are Tapping targets. Tap through each one individually until the emotional charge has decreased significantly or vanished altogether.

Let's look at the process in more detail next. While I'll use a coach as my first example, keep in mind that this Tapping process can be used to understand and navigate many different types of relationship challenges.

Child Tapping: Releasing Angst over a Critical Coach

As one example, let's say your child is struggling with a coach who's asking him/her to practice more, play better and contribute more to the team overall.

To begin, ask your child to tap through the points as you ask these 3 questions one by one, allowing enough time in between for your child to answer each question:

- Is there an encounter with Coach that stands out?
  *Your child's answer points to an **event or remark** that s/he needs to tap on.*

- How do you feel when you think about Coach (and/or that event with Coach)?
  *Your child's answer to this question is the primary **emotion** s/he will use Tapping to release.*

- What do you say to yourself when you're around Coach?
  *Your child's answer may highlight **beliefs** that s/he needs to tap on.*

For example:

Based on the above questions, your child might first share a memory of a recent practice when Coach told him/her that s/he was failing the team.

  ° This is the *event* to tap on.

Your child may then share that s/he feels angry with Coach for saying that.

  ° This is the *emotion* to tap on.

Your child may then share that s/he feels like s/he's never good enough for Coach. No matter how hard s/he practices and plays, Coach is always on him/her to do and be more.

- ° "I am not good enough for Coach" is the *belief* to tap on.

In that case, you might begin by Tapping on the emotion and event, which might look something like this:

Karate Chop *(Repeat 3 times)*: Even though I'm so angry about Coach telling me I'm failing the team, I love myself and accept how I feel.

Eyebrow: So angry

Side of Eye: How could he say that to me?

Under Eye: I've been playing so hard!

Under Nose: I've been to every practice

Under Mouth: How could he say that to me?

Collarbone: I didn't deserve that!

Under Arm: So angry right now!

Top of Head: All this anger

Eyebrow: This hot, burning anger

Side of Eye: I can let myself feel this anger now

Under Eye: I'm never good enough for Coach

Under Nose: That makes me feel so sad

Under Mouth: I've been trying really hard

Collarbone: Sad and angry right now!

Under Arm: I'm not a failure

Top of Head: So angry at Coach right now

Eyebrow: I am NOT a failure and I am NOT failing the team

Side of Eye: All this anger

Under Eye: All this sadness

Under Nose: I can let it all go now

Under Mouth: I don't have to be perfect to be valuable

Collarbone: I don't have to be perfect to be valuable to the team

Under Arm: Letting all this anger and sadness go now

Top of Head: I can relax and feel safe when I think about Coach

Take a deep breath together, and check in with your child on how s/he feels now about Coach. Keep Tapping until s/he gets the desired relief.

Child Tapping: **Releasing Resistance toward a Teacher**

If your child is struggling with a teacher, follow the process outlined in the previous example, **Releasing Angst over a Critical Coach**. That will help you to figure out if the tension between your child and his/her teacher began with a specific event, a communication breakdown, or something else. If your child is upset by a specific event with his/her teacher, such as a teacher reprimanding him/her, tap with him/her on that event, using the "Tell the Story" technique (see page 103 for details).

If your child is suffering from ongoing challenges in a teacher-student dynamic, first try to allow him/her to talk honestly and openly about his/her experiences and feelings without judgment.

Ongoing challenges in relationships with a teacher can sometimes become a source of shame, leading your child to believe that s/he isn't good enough, smart enough, and so on. In that case, you may want to begin by Tapping on those beliefs and emotions.

If your child is struggling to vocalize how s/he feels, you may want to offer prompts, such as:

My teacher makes me feel...

When I'm with my teacher, I feel like...

My teacher thinks I'm...

Once you're clear on how your child is feeling, you can begin Tapping with him/her. That might look something like this:

Karate Chop *(Repeat 3 times)*: Even though I feel like I'm never good/smart/etc. enough for my teacher, I'm still awesome and I'm okay.

Eyebrow: I'm never good enough

Side of Eye: This teacher is always on me

Under Eye: I'm never enough for this teacher

Under Nose: Even when I try hard

Under Mouth: This teacher is always on me

Collarbone: I'm never enough for this teacher

Under Arm: It makes me so mad!

Top of Head: I'm never enough for him/her

Eyebrow: It hurts

Side of Eye: It makes me feel sad

Under Eye: It makes me feel like I'm not enough

Under Nose: So sad about this

Under Mouth: It makes me feel like I'm not enough

Collarbone: It's okay to feel this sadness

Under Arm: It's a feeling

Top of Head: It's not who I am

Eyebrow: This teacher and I are having a hard time

Side of Eye: I don't understand why I'm never enough

Under Eye: Maybe we're just having a hard time understanding each other

Under Nose: It's not my fault

Under Mouth: I can do lots of great things!

Collarbone: This teacher and I don't understand each other

Under Arm: I'm still awesome, though!

Top of Head: I can feel good about myself now

Take a deep breath together and check in with your child on how s/he feels now about his/her teacher. Keep Tapping until s/he gets the desired relief.

Child Tapping: Releasing Anger at a Parent/Guardian

When your child is angry with you or another parent/guardian, it's important first to let them feel that anger. As unsettling as it can be, anger is a natural part of relationships. If you're struggling with your child's anger, be sure to tap on your own feelings about your child's anger first, before Tapping with your child.

Know also that your child may not want to tap when s/he is angry. At that moment s/he may need space. Later, if your child is willing to tap on releasing any remaining anger s/he is feeling, s/he may want to tap without you.

Whether your child taps with or without you, here are some Tapping rounds to get started:

Karate Chop *(Repeat 3 times)*: Even though I feel all this anger and I can feel it in my body, too, I'm okay.

Eyebrow: All this anger

Side of Eye: I can still feel it

Under Eye: It's in my body

Under Nose: I can feel this anger

Under Mouth: All this anger

Collarbone: This big, hot anger

Under Arm: It's in my body

Top of Head: All this anger

Eyebrow: It's okay to feel this anger

Side of Eye: This big, hot anger

Under Eye: It's in my body

Under Nose: It's okay to feel this anger

Under Mouth: I can start to let it go now

Collarbone: I can feel it and then let it go

Under Arm: Letting go of this anger now

Top of Head: Letting myself feel calmer in my body

Eyebrow: Letting myself feel calmer in my mind

Side of Eye: Releasing this anger now

Under Eye: I can relax my body now

Under Nose: And calm my mind

Under Mouth: Releasing this anger now

Collarbone: Feeling calm in my body now

Under Arm: Feeling calm in my mind now

Top of Head: Letting myself relax and feel quiet now

Take a deep breath together, and check in with your child on how angry s/he feels now. Keep Tapping until s/he gets the desired relief.

Since relationships are dynamic, be sure to return to this Tapping process whenever old or new challenges arise.

TAPPING WITH YOUR CHILD: YOUNG LOVE—CRUSHES, FLIRTATION AND HEARTACHE

Crushes, flirtation and heartache—they're natural, normal parts of growing up, but also possible sources of emotional overwhelm. Fortunately, Tapping is a great way to process and release the many emotions children feel as a result of "young love."

As always, the best place to start is by Tapping on your own stress and emotions first, so that you can be fully present when you do tap with your child.

Adult Tapping: **Releasing Stress around Your Child's "Young Love" Experience**

Take a moment to notice how you're feeling about your child's experience around "young love."

Are you less than thrilled about the object of your child's affection? Worried that s/he will feel unworthy after being rejected?

Notice what comes to mind and how you feel about it.

Once you're clear on the primary emotion you're feeling about the situation—worry, anger, sadness, anxiety, etc.—rate that emotion on a scale of 0 to 10.

I'll focus on feelings of anxiety and overwhelm, but as always, tailor your Tapping to how you're feeling.

Take a deep breath and begin by Tapping 3 times on the Karate Chop point:

Karate Chop *(Repeat 3 times)*: Even though I feel so anxious and overwhelmed by this, I love myself and accept how I feel.

Eyebrow: Feeling so overwhelmed

Side of Eye: So anxious

Under Eye: Not sure I'm ready for this

Under Nose: So much anxiety about what my child is going through

Under Mouth: So worried about how s/he's feeling

Collarbone: Not sure how to handle this

Under Arm: It's hard to talk about this with him/her

Top of Head: I'm not sure how to handle all of this

Eyebrow: I'm not sure what to do or not do

Side of Eye: It's overwhelming

Under Eye: And I feel anxious about it

Under Nose: All this anxiety and overwhelm

Under Mouth: I can let myself feel it all now

Collarbone: Maybe there are no answers

Under Arm: Maybe I can focus on feeling these emotions

Top of Head: I can first accept how I'm feeling now

Eyebrow: And then let it all go

Side of Eye: Releasing this anxiety and overwhelm

Under Eye: Releasing it from my mind and body now

Under Nose: It's okay to feel these feelings

Under Mouth: And it's safe to let them go now

Collarbone: Releasing these feelings from every cell in my body now

Under Arm: Allowing myself to feel calm and peaceful about this situation

Top of Head: Feeling quiet and calm now

Take a deep breath and rate your primary emotion(s) again. Keep Tapping until you get the desired relief.

Now that you've had an experience, let's look at how to tap with your child on some of the common emotions that arise as a result of "young love."

Note: As always, when Tapping with your child, tailor your words to your child's age and experience.

"I Don't Want to Kiss You!"

Some children experiment with "young love" feelings and behaviors earlier than others. These different developmental timelines can cause confusion, even friction, between children who were once the best of friends.

That was the case for Ruby, who was having a great time in kindergarten. In addition to bonding with her teacher, she had become close friends with her classmate, Robert. They played often and well, both in school and during playdates.

One day during a playdate at Ruby's house, Robert asked her to kiss him on the lips. Ruby responded, "Maybe when we're older, but not now."

When Ruby told her mom later that afternoon about Robert's request, Ruby seemed calm but slightly bothered. Aware that Robert had two teenage siblings, both of whom were in relationships, Ruby's mom knew that Robert was copying his older siblings. Still, though, she wasn't sure what to do to help Ruby process her feelings.

A few weeks later, the school year ended. Since Robert was moving to a new town over the summer, that also meant saying goodbye to him. When Ruby's mother asked how she was feeling about Robert leaving, she shared that she had mixed feelings. Having him as a friend had been really fun, but she still felt uncomfortable about his request for a kiss.

Ruby's mom asked if she wanted to tap about it. Ruby nodded yes. As they tapped through the points, Ruby shared that she was angry that Robert had asked her for a grown-up kiss. They tapped on feeling and then releasing her anger. Very quickly, Ruby became noticeably more relaxed. By the end of their Tapping, Ruby was calm and happy.

Since Tapping that day, Ruby has been able to remember Robert fondly, rather than as the boy who asked for a kiss.

While I love the immediate results in stories like Ruby's, I also often think about the future benefits of Tapping like this. After years of Tapping with adults who suffer from repressed emotions related to childhood events, I can't help but wonder how this simple Tapping on Robert's kiss might transform Ruby's future. In the years to come, once she is sincerely ready for her first grown-up kiss, she may feel genuinely excited, rather than fearful and resistant. That alone could positively transform her entire adult experience around physical intimacy and relationships.

Younger Child Tapping: Releasing Icky Feelings about Unwanted Attention/Affection

If your child, like Ruby, is struggling with emotions about requests to express unwanted attention or affection, ask him or her how s/he is feeling—mad, sad, icky, etc.

Ask your child to rate that emotion, either on a scale of 0 to 10 or using the "this much" method of measurement.

As always, use your child's words and experience as you tap with him/her.

Take a deep breath together and begin by Tapping 3 times on the Karate Chop point.

Karate Chop (*Repeat 3 times*): Even though I feel so icky about this, I'm a great kid and I'm okay.

Eyebrow: I feel icky about this

Side of Eye: I don't like it

Under Eye: It feels icky

Under Nose: It's okay to feel this way

Under Mouth: I'm safe

Collarbone: I'm a great kid!

Under Arm: And I'm okay

Top of Head: I can let this feeling go now

Eyebrow: I'm safe

Side of Eye: And I can let this go

Under Eye: I'm a great kid

Under Nose: And I'm okay

Under Mouth: I can say "no" when I don't like something

Collarbone: I'm safe, even when I say "no"

Under Arm: I'm okay

Top of Head: And I'm a great kid!

Eyebrow: I can feel calm and safe now

Side of Eye: I can feel okay now

Under Eye: I'm a great kid!

Under Nose: And I'm okay

Under Mouth: I can feel good now

Collarbone: I'm a great kid!

Under Arm: And I'm okay

Top of Head: Feeling calm and quiet inside now

Take a deep breath together and ask your child to rate his/her emotion(s) again. Keep Tapping until s/he gets the desired relief.

"S/he Won't Leave Me Alone!"

Issues around "young love" often become more challenging as children approach middle school. During these years, children are often more physically mature than they are emotionally and mentally mature, which can add to confusion and emotional overwhelm.

Anna's 10 year-old daughter, Lorelei, was in the throes of that overwhelm at bedtime one night. Sensing that something was off, Anna asked her if she wanted to talk.

Lorelei shared that she was frustrated about a boy in her class who wouldn't leave her alone. He wasn't hurting her or even being mean, but he was constantly seeking out her attention, and it had become annoying. To make matters worse, she'd asked him to stop bothering her, but he'd ignored her request and continued anyway.

As she described how he was pestering her, Lorelei's voice and demeanor became panicked. She felt like there was nothing she could do to stop this boy from bothering her.

Knowing that her daughter would say no if she outright asked her to tap, Anna began Tapping, and invited her daughter to follow along, *if* she wanted to. To Anna's surprise and delight, Lorelei followed her mom's lead and tapped through the points alongside her.

They began with a setup statement about the frustration she was feeling about this boy bugging her at school constantly, and then moved through the points, using phrases like:

He won't leave me alone

It frustrates me

It makes me uncomfortable

I feel overwhelmed

I tried to tell him to stop

He didn't listen

This feeling of frustration

After one round of Tapping, Lorelei was transformed. Looking relaxed and peaceful, she took a deep breath, smiled, and shared that she was feeling much better. She then gave her mom a big hug, got in bed, and quickly fell asleep.

Although she uses Tapping herself, Anna was amazed at how quickly Tapping had calmed her daughter. Usually when Lorelei was upset, they'd spend 20 or more minutes discussing and reviewing what had happened before she could calm down enough to go to sleep. This night, thanks to Tapping, their entire talking/Tapping took only 10 minutes. Plus, Lorelei had relaxed far more deeply, and in half the time, than she ever had before by just talking!

One of my favorite parts of this story is the way Anna gave Lorelei the option to join in and tap with her. By age 10, kids are already beginning to avoid "weird" things, especially from their parents. Anna's solution was simple, wise and empowering. Love it!

Child Tapping: Releasing the Stress of Unwanted Attention

If your child is receiving unwanted attention, ask him/her how s/he feels about it. If possible, focus on one or two primary emotion(s).

Ask him/her to rate the intensity of that emotion(s), either on a scale of 0 to 10 or using the "this much" method of measurement.

Take a deep breath together and begin by Tapping 3 times on the Karate Chop point.

Karate Chop *(Repeat 3 times)*: Even though I feel uncomfortable and overwhelmed by all this attention, I love myself and accept how I feel.

Eyebrow: This attention

Side of Eye: It's too much

Under Eye: It's overwhelming

Under Nose: I don't like it

Under Mouth: It makes me so uncomfortable

Collarbone: I just want things to feel normal again

Under Arm: I don't like all this attention

Top of Head: It's overwhelming

Eyebrow: And frustrating

Side of Eye: It won't stop

Under Eye: I don't like it

Under Nose: I feel frustrated and overwhelmed by this attention

Under Mouth: It's okay for me to feel that way

Collarbone: I'm safe and I can relax when I think about it

Under Arm: I still don't like it, though

Top of Head: I can ask <name> to respect my wishes

Eyebrow: I'm a great kid!

Side of Eye: I can relax about this

Under Eye: And ask <name> to stop when I feel uncomfortable

Under Nose: It's okay to say "no" when it feels right

Under Mouth: I'm safe and I can relax now

Collarbone: I can relax and feel calm now

Under Arm: And let go of this overwhelmed feeling

Top of Head: Letting myself feel quiet and calm now

Take a deep breath, and ask your child to rate his/her primary emotion(s) again. Keep Tapping until s/he gets the desired relief.

Pre-Teen/Teenager Tapping: Quieting Obsessive Thoughts about a Crush

If your child is on the other end of the equation and is feeling overwhelmed by a crush s/he has on someone else, Tapping can help him/her to feel calmer and more at ease with the crush.

Note: Awakening to "young love" is often a sensitive topic. Feeling obsessed—including having a hard time focusing—due to a crush is a normal, healthy part of growing up. Using Tapping to "fix" your child's feelings or lack of focus may cause them to feel shame around having an intense crush, even when your intention is simply to help him/her to relax. As always, let your child drive the process. As one example, if your child is expressing frustration about the crush s/he has, you might suggest Tapping as a way to feel less frustrated. If your child seems obsessed but not frustrated by it, it may be best to let them have that experience and instead use Tapping to process and release your own worry, stress and so on.

First ask your child to focus on the crush s/he has and how s/he feels about it. When s/he is clear on the primary emotion(s)—frustration, anxiety, nervousness, etc.—ask him/her to rate the feeling, either on a scale of 0 to 10 or using the "this much" method of measurement.

I'll use frustration as the primary emotion, but as always, tailor your words to your child's experience.

Take a deep breath together and begin by Tapping 3 times on the Karate Chop point.

Karate Chop *(Repeat 3 times)*: Even though I feel so frustrated, and I can't stop thinking about <name>, I love myself and accept how I feel.

Eyebrow: So frustrating!

Side of Eye: Can't stop thinking about <name>

Under Eye: I can't relax

Under Nose: All I do is think about <name>!

Under Mouth: It's exciting

Collarbone: And kind of fun sometimes

Under Arm: But it's also annoying!

Top of Head: And it makes it hard to relax

Eyebrow: My mind won't stop

Side of Eye: Always thinking about <name>

Under Eye: It's fun, but also hard to relax

Under Nose: That's okay

Under Mouth: It's okay to feel this way

Collarbone: Maybe I can let myself relax a little bit

Under Arm: And let go of this frustration

Top of Head: It's hard to stop thinking about <name>

Eyebrow: And that's okay

Side of Eye: I can enjoy it

Under Eye: And let go of this frustration

Under Nose: I can let myself feel more relaxed

Under Mouth: And focus on other things when I choose to

Collarbone: Releasing this frustration now

Under Arm: Letting myself relax

Top of Head: Allowing myself to feel calm and quiet now

Take a deep breath together, and check back in with your child on how intense his/her primary emotion is now. Keep Tapping until s/he gets the desired relief.

Healing from Heartbreak

Heartbreak is an overwhelming experience for everyone, especially for children/teenagers who are newer to the experience and unsure of how to handle and heal their shattered hearts. Thankfully, Tapping supports faster and more complete emotional release.

Dave, 17 years old, hurt deeply after his longtime girlfriend unexpectedly broke up with him. Her departure had shocked him and left him with feelings of overwhelming sadness. To intensify his distress, she had broken up with him at the start of a new school year, when he was surrounded by friends who had long known them as a couple.

Hoping to support him through his heartbreak, Dave's mother, who had tapped with him previously, asked him if he wanted to tap. He promptly agreed, and they did several rounds on his shock and sadness. As they were Tapping, Dave began to cry, sharing that he felt like he'd been abandoned again, which is what his father had done when Dave was in elementary school. It was a deep emotional wound from a decade earlier that hadn't yet healed.

Over a period of days, Dave continued to cry, letting himself feel, and then release, a sadness that had felt bottomless, bigger and more intense than he thought he could handle.

After a week, though, he woke up one morning as his former self. There was a sparkle in his eye, and no hint of the sadness he'd allowed himself to release. Dave has since used Tapping on issues with friends, sports injuries, as well as physical pain. Most important of all, thanks to Tapping he is releasing repressed emotions and building positive self-esteem, focusing on self-love rather than on the kid who was abandoned by his dad.

Pre-Teen/Teenager Tapping: "S/he Dumped Me"

Often the first pain point of a breakup is the breakup event itself. Sometimes the way a breakup happens—via text, social media or email—stings the worst.

Other times, it's what the person did or didn't say—or something else altogether—that may hurt the most.

To begin, let your child talk through what happened and how s/he is feeling.

For the purpose of this exercise, try not to sympathize, justify or judge his/her experience or emotions. This is a clearing exercise, so it's also best to avoid sharing your own stories and wisdom. Instead, just listen as your child speaks.

If your child is willing to tap, ask what primary emotion(s) s/he is feeling around the breakup event, and ask him/her to rate the intensity of that emotion on a scale of 0 to 10.

Next, use the "Tell the Story" technique:

As you both tap through the points, listen while your child tells the story of the breakup event.

When s/he gets to the first point of emotional intensity, gently ask him/her to pause and rate the emotional intensity of that specific point in the story. Tap through that one moment in the story until it holds little to no emotional charge.

Once that moment has been neutralized, ask your child to return to the beginning of the story. Have him/her tell the story until s/he reaches a second point of emotional intensity.

Again, tap only on that moment until its emotional charge is nearly or completely gone.

Ask your child to begin the story from the beginning again and tell it until s/he reaches a third point of emotional intensity. Use Tapping to neutralize that moment and retell the story from the beginning.

Continue repeating this process until your child can tell his/her breakup story from start to finish without experiencing an emotional charge.

Note: For a complete description of the "Tell the Story" technique, see page 103.

Keep in mind that even after neutralizing the breakup event, your child may still feel challenging emotions around the breakup itself, as well as other events, people and places related to the now broken relationship. This exercise is a first step in what may be a longer process.

Once the breakup event has been neutralized, if your child is willing, you can focus your Tapping on releasing specific emotions, such as anger, sadness, or whatever s/he is feeling, as well as any other events and beliefs related to his/her breakup.

Pre-Teen/Teenager Tapping: "I Don't Want to Talk about It"

If your child seems to be suffering after a breakup or rejection, but isn't willing to talk about it, ask if s/he is willing to try a little bit of Tapping that might help him/her to feel better. Reassure him/her that s/he won't have to talk about what s/he is feeling.

Take a deep breath together, and begin by Tapping 3 times on the Karate Chop point:

Karate Chop *(Repeat 3 times)*: Even though I don't want to talk about it, I'm okay.

Eyebrow: I don't want to talk about it

Side of Eye: I don't want to talk about it

Under Eye: I don't even want to think about it

Under Nose: That's okay

Under Mouth: I don't have to talk about it

Collarbone: It's hard not to think about it, though

Under Arm: I don't want to talk about this

Top of Head: That's okay

Eyebrow: I don't have to talk about this

Side of Eye: I'm not even sure what I feel

Under Eye: I feel a lot of things

Under Nose: It's too much to think about

Under Mouth: I don't want to talk about this

Collarbone: That's okay

Under Arm: I don't have to talk about this

Top of Head: I can let myself relax now

Eyebrow: I can let this all go now

Side of Eye: It's not fun

Under Eye: I don't like it

Under Nose: It's too much

Under Mouth: That's okay

Collarbone: I can relax now anyway

Under Arm: This isn't who I am

Top of Head: And I can relax and feel safe now

Take a deep breath together and keep Tapping until your child gets the desired relief. Whether or not s/he chooses to share more about what happened and how s/he is feeling, trust that even a little bit of Tapping can allow for healing to begin. As always, if you're struggling to trust that, tap on it!

Pre-Teen/Teenager Tapping: Releasing Big Emotions around Breakup/Rejection

If your child is feeling emotional about a breakup or rejection, ask him/her to notice his/her primary emotion(s) and rate its emotional intensity on a scale of 0 to 10.

I'll focus on sadness, but if your child is feeling angry, jealous, regretful, or anything else, tailor your Tapping, as always, to what s/he is feeling.

Take a deep breath together and begin by Tapping 3 times on the Karate Chop point.

Karate Chop *(Repeat 3 times)*: Even though I feel all this sadness, and it's so overwhelming, I'm okay.

Eyebrow: So much sadness

Side of Eye: All this sadness

Under Eye: It feels bigger than me

Under Nose: It feels devastating

Under Mouth: So much sadness

Collarbone: How did this happen?

Under Arm: All this sadness

Top of Head: So much sadness

Eyebrow: It's okay to feel it now

Side of Eye: It hurts

Under Eye: So much sadness

Under Nose: It's overwhelming

Under Mouth: I can let myself feel it now

Collarbone: Even though it hurts

Under Arm: It's safe to feel it all now

Top of Head: It hurts, but I'm okay

Eyebrow: It's safe to feel this now

Side of Eye: And safe to let it go now

Under Eye: I can feel this sadness

Under Nose: And I can let it go

Under Mouth: It's safe to let it go

Collarbone: Even though it feels like such a big ending

Under Arm: I can feel safe letting it go now

Top of Head: Letting myself relax and feel safe now

Take a deep breath together and check in on how your child is feeling. Keep Tapping until s/he gets the desired relief.

Pre-Teen/Teenager Tapping: "What Will They Think?"

At this age, relationships may be intimately related to larger social circles that have a big impact on your child's identity and social life.

If your child is concerned about how a breakup or rejection will impact his/her social life in a broader sense, ask him/her first to notice what emotion s/he is feeling most intensely. Is s/he worried about being rejected by a larger group due to a breakup or rejection? Afraid of what people will think of him/her because of a breakup or rejection? Angry or sad that others knew something before s/he did?

Once your child is clear on his/her primary emotion(s), ask him/her to rate its intensity on a scale of 0 to 10.

As always, whenever possible, use your child's words when you're Tapping together.

Take a deep breath and begin by Tapping 3 times on the Karate Chop point.

Karate Chop *(Repeat 3 times)*: Even though I'm so worried about how everyone will react, I'm okay.

Eyebrow: What will they think?

Side of Eye: How will they react?

Under Eye: So stressful

Under Nose: The breakup is bad enough!

Under Mouth: Don't need this

Collarbone: But still, I'm stressed out

Under Arm: What will they think?

Top of Head: Will we still all be friends?

Eyebrow: Will we still all hang out?

Side of Eye: Not sure how I feel about all this

Under Eye: It's overwhelming

Under Nose: I'm stressed about it

Under Mouth: How everyone will react

Collarbone: Feels so awkward

Under Arm: This sucks

Top of Head: I hate this!

Eyebrow: It's okay to let myself feel this

Side of Eye: Even though it feels overwhelming

Under Eye: Letting myself feel all of this now

Under Nose: And letting it all go now

Under Mouth: I can let things unfold one day at a time

Collarbone: I'm safe letting this all go now

Under Arm: I can let myself relax and feel safe about this

Top of Head: It's safe to feel safe and trust that things will work out

Take a deep breath together. Check with your child on the intensity of his/her emotion(s) now. Keep Tapping until s/he gets the desired relief.

Pre-Teen/Teenager Tapping: Moving On after Heartbreak

During the heartbreak healing process, small moments— seeing an old photo of an ex, walking by the spot where they shared something, or even a remark from a well-meaning friend, can trigger intense and challenging emotions. This simple but powerful exercise can help your child to let go of those emotionally charged moments, and move on in a healthier way.

First ask your child to focus on the moment that has triggered him/her. Keep in mind, for this exercise, s/he needs to focus on a brief moment, such as seeing an ex flirting with someone else, or walking by a spot that holds memories that now cause pain.

Note: If there are several moments, tap through each one individually. If the moments are all connected parts of a single story, use the "Tell the Story" technique (see page 103 for details).

To begin, ask your child to focus his/her attention on that single moment and notice what emotion(s) s/he feels most intensely when s/he focuses on that. Ask him/her to rate the intensity of that emotion on a scale of 0 to 10.

Take a deep breath, and begin Tapping while your child replays the moment over and over again, either out loud or silently in his/her mind.

For instance, if your child is obsessing about seeing his/her ex flirting with someone else, s/he should focus just on that moment.

Ask your child to tap through the points while either talking out loud or simply replaying the moment over and over again in his/her mind.

Then ask him/her again what emotion(s) s/he feels when focusing on that moment.

Tap through that emotion, using simple phrases like:

For regret:

This regret... I should have been around more... I should have been there for him/her... All this regret...

For jealousy:

This jealousy... this intense jealousy... why isn't it me...? All this jealousy...

Keep Tapping through the emotion until its charge is either gone or greatly diminished.

Then, as your child continues to tap through the points, replay the moment from start to finish. Tap through any remaining emotional charge until your child can recall the moment without feeling emotional intensity.

To finish, do at least one—or several—positive rounds of Tapping, which might look something like this:

Karate Chop *(Repeat 3 times)*: Even though this breakup really happened, and it's been hard to get through, I'm going to be all right.

Eyebrow: This breakup

Side of Eye: It's been really painful

Under Eye: So many memories and moments

Under Nose: I've had a lot to tap through

Under Mouth: That's okay

Collarbone: That's what happens after breakups

Under Arm: It's okay for me to feel all of these things

Top of Head: And it's okay for me to let them go

Eyebrow: This breakup wasn't my fault

Side of Eye: This breakup happened

Under Eye: But it's not who I am

Under Nose: It's really hurt

Under Mouth: But it doesn't define me

Collarbone: I can feel all of my feelings

Under Arm: And feel safe letting them go

Top of Head: It's hard to move on

Eyebrow: It's hard to let go all the way

Side of Eye: Part of me wants to hold on still

Under Eye: But it's time to really let go

Under Nose: It's time for a new chapter to begin

Under Mouth: And it's safe to let that happen

Collarbone: I can feel excited about this new chapter

Under Arm: And feel safe and relaxed

Top of Head: Letting myself feel safe and calm now

Keep Tapping until your child can feel this positive energy about his/her new chapter, and return to this exercise whenever it seems helpful.

Chapter 14

Overcoming Personal Challenges

TAPPING WITH YOUR CHILD: "BIG T" AND "LITTLE T" TRAUMA

In this section we'll look at how to use Tapping on two different kinds of trauma—"little t" trauma and "Big T" trauma. We've talked a lot about trauma and how it can manifest in the previous chapters, but here we'll go into it in more specific detail.

"Little t" TRAUMA

While the word *trauma* is commonly associated with major, life-altering, "Big T" trauma events, multiple "little t" traumas can also have a profound cumulative impact on health and wellness.

Most people, including those with fulfilling lives and happy childhoods, have experienced "little t" traumas, which span a huge range of experiences, from bullying to just losing something, or many other isolated instances. As just one example, if as a child you were temporarily lost in a crowd one day, that event and the fear it caused may constitute a "little t" trauma.

What often happens is, without our conscious awareness, post-traumatic stress accumulates over time. Similar to the way a glass eventually overflows if we continue to pour water into it, multiple "little t" and/or "Big T" traumas, even when they occur over a span of many years, will eventually cause our internal "glass" to overflow. That's why "little t" trauma experienced in childhood often doesn't manifest through physical or emotional symptoms until adulthood—it took all those years in between for that person's internal "glass" to overflow.

Until you create more space within your internal "glass," which you can do by Tapping on releasing current as well as past trauma, you remain stuck, unable to heal or move forward.

As parents, of course, we want nothing more than to keep our children's internal "glass" empty and trauma-free. Just considering the possibility that our children may have experienced some form of trauma is traumatic unto itself.

Before we look at using Tapping with your child on their "little t" trauma, let's do some Tapping on releasing your own emotions first.

Adult Tapping: **Releasing the Stress of Your Child's Experience**

Take a moment to focus on what your child has experienced. Whether you know s/he has undergone "little t" trauma, or just fear that s/he may have, what emotion(s) comes up most intensely when you focus on it—fear, anger, regret or something else?

Notice what comes up and rate the intensity of your primary emotion(s) on a scale of 0 to 10.

Take a deep breath and begin by Tapping 3 times on the Karate Chop point.

Karate Chop *(Repeat 3 times)*: Even though I'm so worried about what my child has experienced, it's too much at this age, I love myself and accept how I feel.

Eyebrow: So worried about her

Side of Eye: So scared about how this will impact her future

Under Eye: So angry this happened

Under Nose: It's my job to protect her

Under Mouth: How did this happen?

Collarbone: She's too young for this

Under Arm: So worried about how this will impact her

Top of Head: So much stress and worry about this

Eyebrow: I'm supposed to protect her

Side of Eye: How did this happen?

Under Eye: I'm so worried about this

Under Nose: So scared about how this will impact her

Under Mouth: All this fear and worry

Collarbone: It's safe to feel it all now

Under Arm: And it's safe to let it all go now

Top of Head: We can get through this

Eyebrow: But I need to feel all of this fear and worry first

Side of Eye: And let it all go now

Under Eye: We can get through this

Under Nose: I can be there to help her through this

Under Mouth: First, I need to release all these emotions

Collarbone: And love and support myself

Under Arm: So I can love and support her

Top of Head: It's safe to let these emotions go now

Take a deep breath and check back in on the stress and worry or other emotion(s) you were feeling. How intense do they feel now? Give them a number on a scale of 0 to 10. Keep Tapping until you get the desired relief.

Now that you've had an experience, let's look at how to use Tapping with your child.

Note: As always, when Tapping with your child, tailor your words to your child's age and experience.

Releasing "Little t" Trauma

During a playdate at her friend's house, Suzie, at 8 years old, witnessed her friend putting her hand in boiling water. Terrified by what had happened in front of her, Suzie began screaming uncontrollably. Her reaction to what she'd seen was so intense, in fact, that by the time the paramedics were done treating the burn, her friend's mother was as concerned about Suzie as she was about her own daughter.

This is a great example of "little t" trauma. Although Suzie herself hadn't been physically harmed, she felt emotionally traumatized from witnessing her friend's burn.

With kids, as well as adults, these "little t" trauma moments can feel incredibly intense. Whether from watching a scary movie, seeing someone get hurt or many other situations, "little t" traumas can lead to long-term fears, phobias, nightmares and more. Because Tapping addresses the trauma on physical, emotional and mental levels, it's a powerful way to neutralize events like this one.

When Suzie's parents arrived at the friend's house, the paramedics were done treating and bandaging her friend's burn. Almost immediately, Suzie's mother began Tapping on her. Within a few minutes of Tapping, Suzie calmed considerably. They then continued to tap together while talking about what happened and how she felt watching her friend in such acute pain. She also shared how she'd felt upon seeing her friend's skin being visibly injured.

Within a few minutes of Tapping, Suzie could discuss the event calmly. She understood that, although the burn had caused her friend pain, the doctors had taken care of her, and she was all right.

Both of Suzie's parents were stunned by how quickly she'd been able to calm down with Tapping. She'd always been highly sensitive and often had trouble calming herself after becoming upset. Since that day, they've used Tapping more often with all of their children.

Suzie's story is a great example of how powerful it is to tap on a traumatic event immediately after it happens. While Tapping can produce powerful healing long afterward as well, Tapping on trauma when the experience is still vivid and real can be especially powerful. Let's look at how to do that now.

Child Tapping: Immediately after a "Little t" Trauma

When a traumatic event is fresh in your child's mind, the most powerful healing gift you can give him/her is your presence. Rather than worrying about what to say or not say, let your child speak while Tapping through the points. Don't worry about rating the intensity of their emotions. Instead, let him or her talk and tap.

This is basically a free-form version of the "Tell the Story" technique (see page 103). As your child taps and says whatever s/he is thinking, feeling or remembering, tap along while giving her or him your full presence. As always, you can also tap on the points for your child if s/he is unable or unwilling.

If at any point your child has trouble verbalizing what s/he is feeling or thinking, s/he can also replay the event in his or her mind while Tapping.

If your child seems stunned or unsure, you can also tap through the points while saying something like, "I feel numb," "I can't think about this," or "What just happened?"

Your goal here is to lower your child's stress as quickly as you can, and then let her or him talk and think through whatever s/he needs to while Tapping.

Continue Tapping until your child can recall the event without experiencing an emotional charge.

Child Tapping: Releasing a Traumatic Memory

If your child is struggling with a past memory of a "little t" trauma, the best starting point is usually the "Tell the Story" technique (see page 103). To begin, gently prompt your child to recall sights, sounds, smells, sensations, what people said and did, and so on as s/he taps.

At each point of emotional intensity in the story, stop and rate the moment or emotion and then tap through just that point in the story until it's been neutralized.

Continue this process until your child can run through the entire story without experiencing an emotional charge.

Now that we've seen how to use Tapping on "little t" trauma, let's look at how Tapping can help you and your child to move beyond "Big T" trauma, which typically has a much deeper and larger impact on well-being.

"Big T" Trauma

Major trauma, which we also call "Big T" trauma, refers to life-altering events such as terrorist acts, loss of loved ones, serious accidents, sexual molestation, natural disasters, chronic neglect, abuse, etc.

When "Big T" trauma strikes, it so often strips us of our most basic sense of peace and security. As the outside world urges us to get back to living, we're continually faced with the fact that the "normal life" we once knew no longer exists. As a result, we often feel isolated exactly when we need love and support the most.

The very real physical and emotional post-traumatic stress that we then experience quickly becomes an ingrained response. Research has shown, in fact, that the brain reorganizes itself after trauma in ways that *increase* stress and *decrease* resilience[1]. As a result, as time passes, post-traumatic stress gets worse.

To disrupt this painful cycle, we have to communicate directly with the amygdala, which is the part of the brain that initiates the stress response in the body. Given that Tapping is a powerful way to send calming signals to the amygdala, it's long been used to alleviate Post-Traumatic Stress Disorder (PTSD) in trauma victims, including military veterans.

While you can experience tremendous relief by Tapping on the symptoms of post-traumatic stress, the key to deep healing is addressing the underlying trauma itself. Given the breadth and depth of "Big T" trauma healing, whenever possible, it's a good idea to work with an EFT practitioner.

At the same time, you can also do a lot of healing work on your own through Tapping. In this section we'll also look at a few stories about how to begin your journey of hope and healing after "Big T" trauma.

Navigating Traumatic Grief

My most personal experiences around "Big T" trauma began on December 14, 2012, when the Sandy Hook Elementary School shooting took place in my hometown of Newtown, CT. On that day, 28 lives were tragically lost, including 20 1st-graders and 6 educators.

Days later, The Tapping Solution Foundation sprang to life. In partnership with my brother Alex, sister Jessica and Dr. Lori Leyden, as well as dozens of volunteer EFT practitioners, I began supporting the countless families, educators, first responders and children devastated by the losses of that day.

A couple of months after we began our work in Newtown, I was asked to visit Scarlett Lewis, whose 6-year-old son, Jesse, had been one of the children tragically lost on that terrible December day. The moment we met, I sensed Scarlett's enormous inner strength. Although devastated by her loss, she hadn't yet given up. Her willingness to even try Tapping was a testament to her incredible courage and faith.

During that first meeting, I asked Scarlett what was bothering her most. She shared that she was angry about something that had happened recently. It was a minor offense, she knew, but she hadn't been able to release her anger toward this person.

Holding onto everyday stressors like this is common in trauma survivors. It's part of the brain's stress response and survival instinct, and also an effective way to avoid facing the larger trauma they've survived.

Once we tapped through her anger around this minor offense, Scarlett could see that by focusing on petty irritations, she was avoiding facing the loss of her beloved Jesse. Over several sessions, we tapped on many other everyday stressors. That eventually paved the way for Tapping on her grief, anger and other deep emotions.

When Scarlett was ready, we also tapped on releasing the emotional charge of the violent and traumatic images that had been haunting her since Jesse's death. During those sessions she also realized that she hadn't yet fully accepted that Jesse was gone. A part of her still held out hope that he was alive, and would one day reappear.

Using Tapping, we were able to peel back the layers of her anger, as well as her overwhelming grief and sadness, which had at times been accompanied by suicidal thoughts.

Through her ongoing process of healing, Scarlett has since felt Jesse's presence in her life once again. Tapping has also helped her to be available to support her older son, JT, in processing his own deep grief.

In the years since, Scarlett has founded the Jesse Lewis Choose Love Foundation, and also written a memoir about her healing journey called *Nurturing Healing Love: A Mother's Journey of Hope & Forgiveness*. She remains a cherished personal friend and someone who continues to inspire me with her tremendous courage and faith in love and healing.

Whether you're dealing with trauma from your own past, or trying to work through trauma that you and your child have survived, it can be incredibly challenging to manage everyday stressors in addition to everything you're going through. Let's do some Tapping on releasing that everyday stress so that you can be more present with your child.

Adult Tapping: Releasing Everyday Stress in the Midst of Trauma

Notice first which everyday stressor(s) really bothers you. Did someone say something upsetting? Are you stressed about money or logistics or some other everyday stressor? Focus on what's bothering you most, and rate its intensity on a scale of 0 to 10.

Take a deep breath, and let's start by Tapping 3 times on the Karate Chop point.

Karate Chop *(Repeat 3 times)*: Even though I'm so stressed about this and I can't let it go, I love myself and accept how I feel.

Eyebrow: So stressed out

Side of Eye: I can't stop thinking about this

Under Eye: All this stress

Under Nose: I can't stop thinking about this

Under Mouth: It's more than I can handle

Collarbone: I shouldn't have to deal with this right now

Under Arm: It's too much

Top of Head: More than I can handle right now

Eyebrow: All this stress

Side of Eye: It's too much

Under Eye: I can't let it go

Under Nose: It's too much

Under Mouth: I can't face what's happened

Collarbone: I can't look at how I'm really feeling

Under Arm: It's not safe

Top of Head: I don't know how to face this

Eyebrow: But I can let myself feel it anyway

Side of Eye: I can let go of these little stresses

Under Eye: And let myself feel these emotions

Under Nose: It's safe to feel my emotions

Under Mouth: I can tap through them

Collarbone: I don't have to do this alone

Under Arm: It's safe to feel all of these emotions

Top of Head: It's safe to feel this now

Take a deep breath and notice how intense your everyday stress feels now. Are you still feeling it, or has your attention shifted to deeper emotions? Rate your stress. Keep Tapping through your experience until you get the desired relief.

Tapping on Traumatic Memories and Images

After trauma people are often haunted by traumatic memories and images. The "Tell the Story" technique is a powerful way to lessen the emotional intensity of these events. For details on that Tapping technique, see page 103 in Chapter 8.

Now that you've had an experience with Tapping, let's look at how to use Tapping with your child after trauma.

Note: As always, when Tapping with your child, tailor your words to your child's age and experience.

Stopping the Spread of The Trauma "Virus"

One of the central tenets of trauma relief work is to understand how quickly trauma can spread. While those at the center of a trauma may be the most severely affected, the larger community typically also suffers from empathetic trauma symptoms that are more subtle and harder to detect.

Keenly aware of how this phenomenon had been playing out in Newtown, CT, since the Sandy Hook Elementary School shooting took place in December 2012, The Tapping Solution Foundation offered a parents' workshop to the larger community.

The group that came together during this workshop was comprised of eleven moms. None of these women knew each other, and none had lost children or been physically present during the shootings. Yet all of them had spent the past two years living in a hypervigilant state, wracked by intense fear, anxiety and survivor's guilt.

For nearly two years all of these women had felt responsible for the lives of their children, husbands, friends and community. They expressed the incredible overwhelm they all felt, as well as the guilt they felt for feeling overwhelmed. They were, after all, the lucky ones, the ones whose families were still intact. Who were they to buckle under a trauma that had affected other families so much more deeply than their own?

One by one, they each expressed that they felt they couldn't let their guards down, because if they did, they would fall apart. If that happened, who would take care of everyone they'd been caring for?

As each parent voiced how she was feeling, Dr. Lori Leyden asked if anyone else could relate to the stories being told. Each time, hands around the room went up. After explaining that these are all common experiences in trauma survivors, the group began Tapping together.

Through Tapping, they began to reconnect with their bodies, and then release the incredible fear, anxiety and guilt that they had been feeling for the previous two years. Finally, they could feel safe in their own bodies again, and let go of the need to try to control everything inside and around them. Instead of trying to survive alone, they could come together and support each other in healing and moving their lives, and the entire community, forward.

"As each person voiced their own truth," Dr. Leyden explained, "they experienced a deep sense of connection with everyone in that room, and realized they weren't alone at all. And that in itself is another miracle."

Whether they're adults or children, trauma survivors often isolate themselves as a way of avoiding additional pain. While that isolation can serve a purpose by helping to keep them safe, over time, as we've seen, that isolation can create additional pain. That's why it's so important to join together with like-minded people and give a voice to what previously seemed unspeakable— traumatic experience, emotions and beliefs—to create a community that supports healthy emotional release and healing from trauma.

Before we begin Tapping on common experiences in trauma survivors, let's look at one more story about post-traumatic stress and how it can manifest.

From Anorexia, Anxiety Disorder & Self-Harm to Recovering from Rape

The long-term effects of "Big T" trauma often manifest through multiple emotional and behavioral symptoms. For Shira, who, at 16 years old, had just arrived at boarding school, those symptoms included an anxiety disorder, anorexia and distorted body image, as well as self-harm and low self-esteem.

Clearly overwhelmed, she began meeting with the school counselor. From their earliest meetings, Shira was open and willing to try Tapping. Within a matter of weeks of beginning to tap, Shira was noticeably less anxious. Her self-esteem also seemed to improve.

Though encouraged by her progress, her counselor remained concerned about Shira's health. In spite of the considerable improvements she'd exhibited since beginning to tap, Shira seemed unable to overcome her anorexia and distorted body image issues. She continued to experience extreme anxiety around eating, and ate very little. As a result, Shira required constant monitoring.

Given Shira's progress in other areas, her counselor felt sure she was missing some essential piece of the story. Wanting to honor and respect Shira's boundaries, she didn't push her to share any more than she was willing.

Nearly two years later, just months before Shira would graduate from boarding school and attend college, Shira shared that she'd been brutally raped when she was 10 years old. Throughout that experience, her rapist had repeatedly told her how fat and ugly she was.

Realizing that Shira had been suffering from PTSD for nearly a decade, the counselor asked Shira if she would be willing to tap on what had happened. Shira agreed, and with her counselor's guidance, began Tapping while telling the story of her rape. Pausing at each point of high intensity to neutralize it before moving forward, Shira shared details of the trauma she'd survived.

As Shira told the story, she repeatedly experienced overwhelming vaginal pain that prevented her from continuing. When that happened, her counselor paused to lead Shira through multiple rounds of Tapping on her vaginal pain. Eventually, the pain would subside enough for Shira to continue Tapping and talking through the event.

After their first Tapping session focusing on her rape, Shira began eating again. Even just by beginning to release the trauma she'd survived, Shira was able to begin nourishing her body.

After the third extended Tapping session focused on her rape, Shira's vaginal pain went away. By the end of their fifth Tapping session focusing on her rape, Shira could tap through the entire story from start to finish. By that point, all of

Shira's trauma symptoms had cleared and her eating had fully stabilized. After years of extreme starvation and suffering, Shira no longer needed monitoring.

It was an incredible transformation that her counselor has continued to follow. Since graduating from boarding school, Shira has been successful academically and has also joined the soccer team. She is thriving and seems very happy.

Many people who have undergone trauma like Shira have multiple issues to address—memories, physical sensations, emotions, beliefs, as well as challenging behavioral patterns that may develop. All of these factors combined can have a profound impact on a trauma survivor's daily experience, as well as that of their loved ones. As you do whatever you can to support your child, make sure to tap on your own stress and emotions. When your child is willing, you can then help him/her to use Tapping to release general, everyday stress.

Due to the complexity of "Big T" trauma, it is recommended, when possible, to seek out a professional who can guide your child through a deeper, more comprehensive trauma healing process. For a list of Certified EFT practitioners, visit http://thetappingsolution.com/eft-practitioners/.

Regaining a Sense of Safety in the Body

One important starting point for overcoming the isolation that trauma survivors often experience is to address a survivor's most basic partnership with his/her own body. After trauma, many survivors lose that sense of being safe in their own skin. Without that most basic trust, they struggle to connect with others.

By using Tapping to foster a greater sense of safety in their own body, trauma survivors can begin a gentle healing process. Let's look next at how to do some general Tapping on that with your child.

Child Tapping: Feeling Safe in Your Body

If your child is willing, have them rate how unsafe they feel in their own body on a scale of 0 to 10 or using the "this much" method of measurement.

Take a deep breath and begin by Tapping 3 times on the Karate Chop point.

Karate Chop *(Repeat 3 times)*: Even though I don't feel safe in my body, I'm a great kid and I'm okay.

Eyebrow: I don't feel safe

Side of Eye: I'm not safe in my own body

Under Eye: Nothing feels the same

Under Nose: I don't feel safe in my own body

Under Mouth: It's hard being around people

Collarbone: And hard being alone

Under Arm: I don't feel safe in my own body

Top of Head: I can't trust that I'm safe

Eyebrow: I don't feel safe in my own body

Side of Eye: Nothing feels the same

Under Eye: I don't feel safe

Under Nose: I don't feel safe in my body

Under Mouth: Too many memories

Collarbone: I'm not safe in my own body

Under Arm: I can't do this

Top of Head: It's too much

Eyebrow: I can take it slowly

Side of Eye: One moment at a time

Under Eye: I'm safe right now

Under Nose: I can take a breath

Under Mouth: I can breathe in

Collarbone: I can breathe out

Under Arm: I can feel safe right now

Top of Head: Letting myself relax in my body now

Keep Tapping on creating a sense of safety. When your child is ready, have him/her share how unsafe s/he feels in his/her body now. Any change, even a small improvement, is a great sign. Trauma healing is a process, so it may take time for your child to experience significant shifts. As always, if your child wants to tap on other issue(s), follow his/her lead, and whenever possible, do more Tapping.

TAPPING WITH YOUR CHILD: DIVORCE

Managing the emotional upheaval and stress of divorce is especially overwhelming when you're also trying to support your children through the transition. While you may feel stressed by the many logistical, financial, practical and emotional issues you're facing, your children may simultaneously be struggling with their own conflicting emotions. The stress that results can make daily life enormously challenging.

Given what a widespread and complex topic divorce is for parents and children alike, we'll take a look at several stories of how parents have used Tapping on themselves, and then introduced Tapping to their children as a way to process and release their many emotions.

To begin, let's take a look at how you, as a parent, can use Tapping to move through the process with more ease and grace.

Announcing Separation/Divorce

After Marta and her husband finalized their decision to separate, she knew it was time to share the difficult news with their 3 children. Their dad would move out of the house soon, and the children needed to know what was happening. On the afternoon when she'd planned to give them the news, however, Marta felt so anxious that she began to feel physically ill.

Recognizing that she needed to calm herself first, Marta closed the door to her room and began Tapping on her panic and nausea, as well as her fear and worry about how her kids would react. She also did some Tapping on a seizing pain she was feeling in her back, along with her intermittent dizziness and a swelling sensation in her throat.

Once her panic as well as her emotional and physical symptoms had sub-sided, she felt calm enough to begin thinking about what she would say to her children. As she continued Tapping through the points, she practiced what she would say, how she would say it, and in what order. She also tapped on the anxi-ety she was feeling about the questions they might ask her, and whether they would blame her for the separation.

An hour later, Marta emerged from her room feeling relatively calm and confident. She then sat down with her children and gently shared the news with understanding and compassion. To her surprise, she didn't feel overwhelmed by her own emotions. Instead, she was able to be present for them during these difficult moments. She listened to them speak, soothed them as they cried, and was able to support them in every way she could without feeling any emotional backlash of her own.

Thanks to Tapping, Marta was able to give her children what they most needed—her full presence.

Let's take a look at how you, too, can use Tapping to feel calmer and more present when you share the news of your divorce with your kids, as well as fam-ily and friends.

Adult Tapping: Announcing Divorce

To begin, find a quiet space where you will be uninterrupted, and take 3 deep breaths. Focus your attention on sharing the news of your divorce with your children.

As you think about it, do a mental scan of your body, and notice how differ-ent parts of your body feel. Is your stomach queasy? Do you feel pain, tightness or clenching anywhere? Do you feel hot or cold anywhere? Any numbness? Try to notice everything you feel in your body.

On an emotional level, what do you feel most intensely—anxiety, dread, anger, fear?

Put all of these together—your emotions and any sensations you feel in your body. How overwhelming does it all feel? Give it a number on a scale of 0 to 10.

Take a deep breath and begin by Tapping 3 times on the Karate Chop point.

Karate Chop *(Repeat 3 times)*: Even though I feel all this overwhelm in my body, heart, and mind, I love myself and accept how I feel.

Eyebrow: So overwhelmed

Side of Eye: I can feel it in my body

Under Eye: I can feel it in my heart

Under Nose: All this overwhelm

Under Mouth: I don't think I can tell them

Collarbone: I don't think I can share this news

Under Arm: So painful to think about

Top of Head: All this overwhelm

Eyebrow: I feel it in my body

Side of Eye: And in my emotions

Under Eye: I can let myself feel it now

Under Nose: I'm not sure I can tell my kids about the divorce

Under Mouth: It's too painful

Collarbone: What if they hate me for it?

Under Arm: Our lives will never be the same

Top of Head: So much overwhelm

Eyebrow: It's okay to feel it now

Side of Eye: Letting myself feel all this overwhelm now

Under Eye: The queasiness in my stomach

Under Nose: The pounding in my head

Under Mouth: I can let myself feel it all now

Collarbone: And I can let it go

Under Arm: I can release this overwhelm

Top of Head: Letting it go now from every cell in my body

Take a deep breath, and notice how overwhelmed you feel now when you think about telling your children about the divorce. Keep Tapping until you get the desired relief.

Next let's look at another intense emotion that parents, as well as children, often experience around divorce—anger.

Releasing Anger after Divorce

Sheila had joined the Parents Group to help her youngest daughter, who, at 15 years old, was suffering from a chronic anxiety disorder. The low point had been over a year earlier, when Sheila's now ex-husband had left. That was when her daughter had stopped functioning. Her unresponsiveness had become so severe that Sheila had been forced to admit her daughter to a mental health facility on a temporary basis.

Her daughter was now home, functioning with the help of a family therapist. Sheila had recently mentioned to the therapist that her daughter would eventually need to talk about her dad because she had unresolved issues around his departure. In response the therapist asked Sheila how she felt about him. Suddenly unable to respond to the therapist's question, Sheila immediately realized that she was still holding onto a great deal of anger toward her ex-husband. She knew that that she would need first to tend to her own emotions before she would be able to help her daughter.

When I asked her to share more, Sheila said that she avoids mentioning her ex-husband altogether. As a single parent, she explained, "You're not supposed to say bad things about the other parent. I don't have many good things to say, so I just don't mention him at all."

During their marriage, he'd assumed the role of stay-at-home dad, leaving Sheila to support the family. It was an arrangement that worked for him, but not for Sheila. He never seemed to care about how she felt, and that had made Sheila feel unsupported. "He was always the victim," she explained. "He blamed me, said I ruined his life, got him fired and made him move back to Portugal."

In cases like these when there are multiple painful memories that hold a high emotional charge, it's helpful to start small and home in on one particular event. When I asked Sheila if anything stood out in her memory, she shared something that had happened a couple of months earlier, after her daughter had returned home.

Her ex had been talking to her son, openly criticizing Sheila for putting their daughter in a facility. Overhearing the exchange, Sheila interrupted the call and told her ex that if he continued to speak badly about her, she'd cut off the call. He replied that he would never forgive her for putting their daughter in a facility. The memory of his remark still infuriated Sheila. He'd been on vacation thousands of miles away when his daughter was suffering most. Once again, he had left her to fend for herself and their children, and then blamed her for the outcome.

Recalling that conversation, Sheila's anger surfaced quickly and easily. To discharge the intensity of her memory, I asked Sheila to begin Tapping as she envisioned that moment. We also tapped on her anger at being expected to support the family and manage their daughter's anxiety issues alone.

As she verbalized her anger, we continued Tapping. After several rounds, she felt calmer. Her anger hadn't dissipated completely, but she was clear on what she needed to do next—tap through her own anger toward her ex-husband. "In this group it seems like an ongoing theme. We all signed up thinking we needed to help our kids, but we really needed to help ourselves first."

At the end of our time together, Sheila agreed to continue Tapping through the anger toward her ex. The anger had decreased, but wasn't yet gone. The difference was that she now knew that she needed to first focus her Tapping on that conversation with her ex. After that, she would need to tap on other events that still made her angry.

By letting go of her own anger, she'd be better able to be available to her two children, who were also trying to recover from their father's absence. Although there was more Tapping to do, her newfound clarity was a source of enormous relief.

Adult Tapping: **Releasing Anger around Divorce**

The best way to begin releasing anger is by focusing on an individual event—one thing that happened, or perhaps one comment your ex-spouse said to you. Even though there may be a long list of events and remarks that make you angry, for now pick only one.

For instance, if you and your ex-spouse had a huge fight and he or she said something that still makes you angry, focus on that. Rate your anger on a scale of 0 to 10.

Take a deep breath and let's begin by Tapping 3 times on the Karate Chop point:

Karate Chop *(Repeat 3 times)*: Even though I feel all this anger when I think about what he/she said to me, I love myself and accept how I feel.

Eyebrow: All this anger

Side of Eye: This red hot anger

Under Eye: So angry right now

Under Nose: All this anger

Under Mouth: I can feel it in my body

Collarbone: How could they say that to me?

Under Arm: "It's all your fault"

Top of Head: "It's all your fault"

Eyebrow: "It's all your fault"

Side of Eye: So angry right now

Under Eye: Those words burn me

Under Nose: I'm not to blame!

Under Mouth: All this anger

Collarbone: It hurts

Under Arm: So much sadness, too

Top of Head. How did this all happen?

Eyebrow: So much anger

Side of Eye: So much sadness

Under Eye: It's too much

Under Nose: I can let myself feel it all, though

Under Mouth: I can let myself feel overwhelmed by it now

Collarbone: And then begin letting it go

Under Arm: Releasing it all now from every cell in my body

Top of Head: Letting this anger and sadness go now

Think again about the comment or event you were Tapping on. When you remember it now, how intense is your anger on a scale of 0 to 10? Keep Tapping until you get the desired relief, and remember to return to this exercise whenever challenging memories or events arise.

Before we look at how to use Tapping with your children, let's look at how to use Tapping to release some of the other common emotions that parents often feel as a result of divorce.

When Peace Seems Impossible

Divorce often introduces an overwhelming amount of upheaval into households. In this story we look at how Tapping can relieve some of that turmoil, and in the process, pave the way for a healthier, gentler transition.

Anita was at her wit's end. Trying to care for her six kids while navigating final divorce proceedings, she was feeling drained by her older son's angry outbursts. The only older boy in the family (Anita's other boy was still a toddler), her son was often contentious and argumentative with his four sisters. He was a great kid, but managing his anger about the divorce had become overwhelming. As much as Anita hated to admit it, the house was often more peaceful when he wasn't home.

With an ex-husband who was still an addict, the majority of her time and energy needed to go toward providing her kids with the stability and nurturing they might never get at their father's house. That by itself was more than a full-time job.

A "tapper" for the past couple of years, Anita had previously tapped with her eldest son, usually before bedtime. To get him to try it, she'd made a deal—she'd do his kitchen chores in exchange for him Tapping with her each night. The results had been more than worthwhile. Whether he'd had a bad day at school or was feeling angry about the divorce, Tapping had seemed to help him get to a calmer place, and then to sleep better, as well. Recently, though, their bedtime Tapping routine had fallen by the wayside.

After hearing about her situation, I asked Anita if her son had recently had an angry outburst, and in fact, just that morning her son had taken his anger out on one of her daughters before school.

Since it's often helpful to begin by Tapping on an issue that still holds an emotional charge, I asked Anita to focus on the events of that morning. I asked her where she could feel the intensity in her body when she thought about how her son provoked her daughter. "I feel a tightness in my chest at about a 7 out of 10," she shared. I asked her what, if any, emotions were contributing to that tightness. She replied that she felt anxiety, frustration and especially guilt. Her guilt was an 8 out of 10.

We did several rounds of Tapping on the tightness in her chest, as well as her frustration, anxiety and guilt. When I paused to ask her how she was feeling, she answered that our Tapping had made her feel "jumbled" or shaken up. As undesirable as that sounds, it's actually encouraging. It means that the Tapping is having an effect. It's hitting different layers of our experience, telling us where to tap next.

We then talked more about her guilt. Did she feel responsible for the end of her marriage? What in particular did she feel guilty about? I gently asked her some questions, hoping to guide her toward more clarity around what she was feeling. She answered that she felt sad that her kids were feeling sad. She was concerned that the divorce was more than they could handle, and that was causing her to feel guilt.

As we continued talking, I asked her to repeat after me, "This is all my fault."

Keep in mind, I didn't actually believe that to be true. Sometimes, however, when we get lost in our emotions, or "jumbled" as she'd described it, it's help-ful to push the boundaries of what feels safe. By forcing ourselves to say what we think we're not supposed to say or think or feel, we may gain much-needed clarity about what we're actually feeling.

When Anita repeated my words, she instinctively shook her head "no" the whole time. The statement didn't resonate with her because she didn't believe that to be true. Her husband was an addict and hadn't wanted to change. She was doing the best she could, making the healthiest decisions possible for herself and her children. That's great! She still may have felt some sadness around her children's sadness, but she realized that guilt didn't fit.

We then did more Tapping on releasing her guilt, and on feeling grounded in her knowing that she was doing the best she could. After several rounds, she shared that she just worried that her son's anger would never end. She was feeling a sense of dread and doom, like she'd never be able to help her son overcome his rage.

We did more Tapping on that feeling of doom. After several rounds, I began Tapping on new possibilities, using reminder phrases like, "What if things could change?" and "What if he could change?" and "What if I could change?" We did several more rounds on opening up to hope that the situation would move forward in positive ways.

"That feels amazing," she commented at one point. "Really Tapping in that sense of hope feels really, really good." We did more rounds on opening up to hope and expanding it.

Anita's story is a great example of how powerful Tapping can be for gaining clarity, which then paves the way for hope and healing to happen. In cases of divorce and other major life events, we often feel so many different emotions that it can be hard to decipher which ones most need our attention.

Adult Tapping: Gaining Clarity

Notice how jumbled, confused and/or overwhelmed you may be feeling as a result of your divorce. Rate the intensity of that confusion on a scale of 0 to 10.

Begin by taking 3 deep breaths. Tap 3 times on the Karate Chop point:

Karate Chop (*Repeat 3 times*): Even though my emotions are all over the place and I'm feeling really jumbled, I deeply and completely love and accept myself.

Eyebrow: All these emotions

Side of Eye: I can't make sense of them

Under Eye: Feeling so jumbled

Under Nose: Just so many emotions around my divorce

Under Mouth: All these emotions I'm feeling

Collarbone: It's really overwhelming

Under Arm: Feeling so jumbled

Top of Head: It's all just too much

Eyebrow: Guilt, overwhelm, anxiety, anger

Side of Eye: So many emotions

Under Eye: They're all hitting me

Under Nose: It's so confusing

Under Mouth: And so overwhelming

Collarbone: I can let myself feel them

Under Arm: I can let myself be overwhelmed by them

Top of Head: It feels like more than I can handle

Eyebrow: But it's really not

Side of Eye: I can let myself feel all of this

Under Eye: And I can let it all go

Under Nose: It's safe to feel all these emotions

Under Mouth: And safe to let them go now

Collarbone: It's safe to feel safe

Under Arm: Even with these emotions in me

Top of Head: Feeling safe with these emotions now

Take a deep breath and notice how intense your confusion is now. Give it a number on a scale of 0 to 10, and keep Tapping until you get the desired relief.

If, through Tapping, you gain further clarity on the other emotions you're feeling, shift your focus to Tapping on those until you get sufficient relief.

Adult Tapping: Releasing Guilt & Shame around Divorce

Guilt is another challenging emotion that often comes up around divorce, especially when children are involved. It's especially important to release guilt ("I *did* a bad thing"), since over time guilt can morph into the deeper, more poisonous emotion that is shame ("I did a bad thing, therefore I *am* a bad person").

To begin, focus on any guilt you may feel around your divorce. For example, if you feel like you failed at marriage and it's hurting your children, rate the guilt you feel on a scale of 0 to 10.

Take a deep breath and let's start by Tapping 3 times on the Karate Chop point:

Karate Chop *(Repeat 3 times)*: Even though I feel so much guilt around the divorce, it's hurting my child so much, I love myself and accept how I feel.

Eyebrow: All this guilt

Side of Eye: I failed at marriage

Under Eye: It's hurting my children

Under Nose: And it's my fault

Under Mouth: All this guilt

Collarbone: What have I done?

Under Arm: How could I let this happen?

Top of Head: Their lives will never be the same

Eyebrow: And it's my fault

Side of Eye: So much guilt

Under Eye: All this guilt

Under Nose: So heavy

Under Mouth: This heavy guilt

Collarbone: It's weighing on me

Under Arm: It's safe to feel this guilt

Top of Head: I can feel it now

Eyebrow: And let it go

Side of Eye: Is it really my fault?

Under Eye: I failed

Under Nose: But really, *we* failed

Under Mouth: Our marriage didn't work

Collarbone: I can let go of this guilt

Under Arm: I can release it now

Top of Head: Allowing myself to let go of this guilt now

Take a deep breath and check back in with your guilt. How intense does it feel now on a scale of 0 to 10? Keep Tapping until you get the desired relief and return to this exercise as often as you need to.

Once the intensity of your own emotional burden has gone down, you'll feel better prepared to tap with your child on how s/he is feeling as a result of the divorce. Let's look at how to do that next.

Note: As always, when Tapping with your child, tailor your words to your child's age and experience.

Releasing Confusion around Mommy vs. Daddy

Deanna had very recently begun divorce proceedings. Her decision to leave had crystallized during a long stretch of time when, due to her husband's work, he had lived out of the country, and more recently, in a different state. Deanna had always been a work-when-she-could mom, available whenever their 3 kids needed her.

Her youngest daughter, Kimberly, who was now in kindergarten, was struggling daily with the news of her parents' divorce. While she was accustomed to her dad being away, the official long-term separation between her parents had felt overwhelming. She was heartbroken that there would be no more excitement about when daddy was coming home.

When Kimberly first learned about her parents' divorce, she had insisted she only wanted to be with her dad. Later, however, she changed her mind, and announced that she only wanted to be with Deanna.

Recognizing Kimberly's confusion, Deanna asked her if she could tap on her one day. When Kimberly nodded yes, she began Tapping through the points on Kimberly while saying, "I really want to be with Mommy" and then, "I really want to be with Daddy," and later, "I'm so confused. I love Mommy and Daddy!" After a couple of rounds, Kimberly nodded, acknowledging the confusion that she was feeling.

A couple of weeks later, Dad came to visit and to pick her up. Overwhelmed by his presence, Kimberly initially threw a fit, exclaiming that she didn't want to leave her mommy. Deanna quietly accompanied Kimberly to her bedroom, telling her ex that they'd quickly finish getting ready.

In the privacy of Kimberly's room, Deanna asked her if she could tap on her. Kimberly nodded yes. Deanna then began Tapping through the points on Kimberly as she voiced her daughter's confusion again. This time, she tailored her Tapping to what was happening at that moment, using phrases like "I really want to stay with Mommy" and "I also want to go with Daddy." After one round of Tapping, Kimberly smiled her biggest smile, and ran out of the room toward her father. "I'm ready! Bye, Mom. See you later!" she exclaimed excitedly.

I love this story because it's such a powerful example of how Tapping can cut through the emotional fog and allow kids, as well as parents, to release the emotions they're feeling. While sharing this story, Deanna, who participated in my Parents Group program, noted that she'd been using Tapping on herself, as well. Tapping had allowed her to be present for her children in challenging moments like these, even though she herself was managing a long list of competing priorities.

Child Tapping: Overcoming Confusion around Choosing a Parent

Since divorce divides Mom and Dad into two different "camps," younger as well as older children may experience confusion around needing to "choose" a parent. That confusion may also create a tendency to blame one parent more than the other for the divorce. Let's look at how to use Tapping to work through that confusion.

Reminder: Be sure to do your own Tapping first, since it's important to respect and honor how your child is feeling, even when their emotions are upsetting to you.

Have your child rate his/her confusion on a scale of 0 to 10, or using the "this much" method of measurement. Then take a deep breath together and start by Tapping on the Karate Chop point.

Karate Chop *(Repeat 3 times)*: Even though I feel confused about the divorce and feel like I need to choose between Mommy and Daddy, I'm a great kid and I'm okay.

Eyebrow: I want to be with Mom

Side of Eye: I want to be with Dad

Under Eye: I want to be with Mom & Dad

Under Nose: I don't like this divorce

Under Mouth: I'm so confused

Collarbone: I love Mommy

Under Arm: And I love Daddy

Top of Head: I don't understand this

Eyebrow: I love Mom

Side of Eye: And I love Dad, too

Under Eye: I don't like this divorce

Under Nose: It's so confusing

Under Mouth: That's okay

Collarbone: I don't have to choose

Under Arm: I can keep loving Mom

Top of Head: And keep loving Dad, too

Eyebrow: Sometimes I can spend time with Dad

Side of Eye: And other times with Mom

Under Eye: I don't have to choose

Under Nose: I can love Mom and Dad

Under Mouth: Things are going to be different

Collarbone: It makes me feel sad

Under Arm: But I'm okay

Top of Head: It's safe to keep loving Mom *and* Dad

Have your child take a deep breath and then measure his/her confusion once again. Keep Tapping until s/he gets the desired relief.

Child Tapping: Releasing Blame & Anger over Divorce

If your child is angry and blames you or your ex-spouse for the divorce, ground yourself by Tapping on your own emotional reactions first.

When you're ready, have your child rate his/her anger and blame, either on a scale of 0 to 10 or using the "this much" method of measurement.

Take a breath and then begin by Tapping 3 times on the Karate Chop point.

Karate Chop *(Repeat 3 times)*: Even though I'm so angry about the divorce, it's all your fault, and I refuse to forgive you, I'm a great kid and I'm okay.

Eyebrow: So angry

Side of Eye: It's your fault

Under Eye: Everything's falling apart

Under Nose: And it's your fault

Under Mouth: So much anger

Collarbone: I hate this divorce

Under Arm: It feels like my whole world is falling apart

Top of Head: So angry

Eyebrow: I blame you for this

Side of Eye: And I won't forgive you

Under Eye: It's your fault

Under Nose: And I'm so angry

Under Mouth: It's safe to feel this anger

Collarbone: And safe to feel this blame

Under Arm: I can let myself feel it all now

Top of Head: And I can let it go

Eyebrow: All this anger

Side of Eye: All this blame

Under Eye: Letting it all go now

Under Nose: It's safe to feel this anger and blame

Under Mouth: And safe to let it all go

Collarbone: I can relax and feel safe now

Under Arm: I don't like this divorce

Top of Head: But I'm a great kid and I'm okay

Take a deep breath and have your child rate the intensity of his/her anger and blame now. Keep Tapping until s/he gets the desired relief. If other emotions arise while Tapping, tap on releasing those as well.

Child Tapping: **Letting Go of Sadness over Divorce**

If your child is feeling sadness about your divorce, begin by having him/her rate that sadness on a scale of 0 to 10 or using the "this much" method of measurement.

Then take a deep breath and begin by Tapping 3 times on the Karate Chop point.

Karate Chop *(Repeat 3 times)*: Even though I feel so sad about my parent's divorce, I'm a great kid and I'm okay.

Eyebrow: Feeling so sad

Side of Eye: How is this even happening?

Under Eye: So sad about this

Under Nose: Everything's falling apart

Under Mouth: This doesn't feel right

Collarbone: All this sadness

Under Arm: It feels so heavy

Top of Head: I can feel it in my body

Eyebrow: All this sadness

Side of Eye: So much sadness

Under Eye: How can this be happening?

Under Nose: So sad about my parent's divorce

Under Mouth: I don't even understand this

Collarbone: It feels so sad

Under Arm: Letting myself feel this sadness now

Top of Head: And letting it go now

Eyebrow: Things will be different

Side of Eye: And that feels sad

Under Eye: It's okay to feel this sadness

Under Nose: It's safe to feel this sadness

Under Mouth: And it's safe to let it go

Collarbone: I can feel this sadness now

Under Arm: And I can let it go now

Top of Head: Releasing this sadness now

Take a deep breath and have your child rate the intensity of his/her sadness now. Keep Tapping until s/he gets the desired relief.

Child Tapping: Adjusting to a New Home

Often at least one parent has to move as a result of divorce. Since that new home is a physical reminder of the separation, your child's first reaction may be to resent and dislike it.

If your child is willing to tap on that resistance, begin by having him or her rate how much s/he dislikes the new home either on a scale of 0 to 10 or using the "this much" method of measurement.

Take a deep breath together and then begin by Tapping 3 times on the Karate Chop point.

Karate Chop *(Repeat 3 times)*: Even though I don't like being here, it's not my home and I don't like it, I'm a great kid and I'm okay.

Eyebrow: I don't like it here

Side of Eye: I don't want to stay here

Under Eye: This isn't my home

Under Nose: And I hate it here

Under Mouth: I don't like it here

Collarbone: It's not my home

Under Arm: It'll never be my home

Top of Head: I want to go back home

Eyebrow: I don't like it here

Side of Eye: I want to go back home now

Under Eye: I don't feel comfortable here

Under Nose: I don't like it here

Under Mouth: Everything's new and it feels weird

Collarbone: I don't like it here

Under Arm: That's okay

Top of Head: I don't have to like it here

Eyebrow: I can relax anyway

Side of Eye: I'm a great kid

Under Eye: And I'm okay

Under Nose: Even though I don't like it here

Under Mouth: It's too new

Collarbone: I can relax and feel safe here anyway

Under Arm: I'm a great kid

Top of Head: And I'm okay here

Take a deep breath together and have your child rate the intensity of his/her dislike of the new home again. Keep Tapping until s/he gets the desired relief.

Child Tapping: Releasing Self-Blame ("My Parents' Divorce Is My Fault")

If your child has taken on the belief that your divorce is his/her fault, first give your child a big hug. If s/he is willing to share, ask why s/he believes this. If, for example, s/he overheard a fight and misinterpreted what s/he heard, make sure to tap on what s/he heard, saw or was told. (For a refresher on Tapping on events, see Chapter 8.)

If her/his belief is a general assumption s/he has made, begin by having her/him rate how true the belief "this divorce is my fault" feels on a 0 to 10 scale or using the "this much" method of measurement.

Take a deep breath and begin by Tapping 3 times on the Karate Chop point.

Karate Chop *(Repeat 3 times)*: Even though I'm so sad because I feel like this divorce is my fault, I'm an awesome kid and I'm okay.

Eyebrow: This divorce

Side of Eye: It's all my fault

Under Eye: I caused problems

Under Nose: And now my parents are divorcing

Under Mouth: It's all my fault

Collarbone: I'm so sad

Under Arm: How could I have done this?

Top of Head: So sad about this divorce

Eyebrow: It's safe to feel this sadness now

Side of Eye: There's so much of this sadness

Under Eye: I feel like it's all my fault

Under Nose: So much sadness in my body

Under Mouth: I can let myself feel it

Collarbone: And I can let it go

Under Arm: Maybe the divorce isn't my fault

Top of Head: Mom and Dad changed and grew apart

Eyebrow: This divorce

Side of Eye: It makes me feel so sad

Under Eye: But it's not my fault

Under Nose: I don't have to feel scared

Under Mouth: I didn't cause this

Collarbone: I can feel safe now

Under Arm: I can feel loved now

Top of Head: Letting myself feel safe and loved now

Take a deep breath together and check back in on your child's belief. How true does it feel now? Keep Tapping until s/he gets the desired relief.

Child Tapping: Accepting a Parent's New Partner

Children often experience a range of overwhelming emotions when one or both parents introduce new partners.

If your child is willing to tap on it, have her/him first share how s/he is feeling. Those feelings may range from anger to sadness, resentment and more.

Next have her/him rate the intensity of her/his primary emotion(s), either on a scale of 0 to 10 or using the "this much" method of measurement.

Take a deep breath together and then begin by Tapping 3 times on the Karate Chop point.

Karate Chop *(Repeat 3 times)*: Even though I don't want this new person in our house, and they're not part of our family, I love myself and accept how I feel.

Eyebrow: I don't like this new person

Side of Eye: He/she is not my parent

Under Eye: And not part of my family

Under Nose: I don't like having him/her around

Under Mouth: I don't want to be friends

Collarbone: I don't want him/her around

Under Arm: He/she isn't part of our family

Top of Head: He/she will never be my parent

Eyebrow: I'm not okay with him/her being around

Side of Eye: It feels like an invasion

Under Eye: I hate how my mom/dad acts around this person

Under Nose: This isn't the way things should be

Under Mouth: I only want my mom and dad

Collarbone: I don't want a stranger in my house

Under Arm: I'm angry about him/her being here

Top of Head: It's okay to feel angry and uncomfortable about this

Eyebrow: It's okay to have these feelings

Side of Eye: I can let myself feel them fully now

Under Eye: This doesn't feel right

Under Nose: Having this new person around doesn't feel comfortable

Under Mouth: It's okay to feel all of this now

Collarbone: And it's safe to let it go

Under Arm: Releasing all these feelings around this new person

Top of Head: Allowing myself to relax and feel safe now

Take a deep breath together and have your child rate the intensity of his/her emotion(s) again. Keep Tapping until s/he gets the desired relief.

We've tapped through several different events, emotions and beliefs related to divorce. If your child is suffering from other issues, such as anxiety, fears or other symptoms like nightmares, refer to those sections, as well as Chapter 9, for additional guidance. Remember, too, that divorce is a process, so tap as often and for as long as you and your child need.

Chapter 15

Healing

TAPPING WITH YOUR CHILD: ALLERGIES & ASTHMA

After years of helping clients relieve their allergy and asthma symptoms with Tapping, I was excited—and a bit shocked!—to find an article from August 28, 1948, in *The Toledo Blade* newspaper linking hay fever and asthma to emotions[1]. The article reported on the results of a study in Beverly Hills, CA, that focused on 22 patients (7 men, 8 women, 7 children). All 22 participants had been treated unsuccessfully with conventional methods. After expressing their emotions, 21 of the 22 patients experienced an improvement in their allergies and asthma.

In the years since, of course, numerous studies have linked allergies and asthma to depression, anxiety, sleep disorders and more.[2] While we don't fully understand how emotions tie into allergies and asthma—for instance, whether anxiety contributes to allergies or results from them—we do know that stress, as well as negative emotions, can weaken the immune system. As a result, anxiety and stress make us more likely to experience severe allergy symptoms as well as asthma attacks.

In this section, we'll look at how to use Tapping to address allergy and asthma symptoms, as well as some of the emotions to which they may be linked. To begin, we'll first do some Tapping on the stress, anxiety and fear you may experience as a result of your child's allergies and asthma.

Safety First! **When using Tapping for asthma and any other potentially life-threatening condition(s), always follow your doctor's advice first and foremost. Rely first on traditional safety measures—from inhalers to calling an ambulance or other—and use Tapping to supplement those measures.**

Adult Tapping: Lowering Allergy- and Asthma-Related Stress

When you think about your child's allergies and/or asthma, what emotion do you feel most intensely—fear, helplessness, anxiety? Give it a number on a scale of 0 to 10.

Take 3 deep breaths, then tap 3 times on the Karate Chop point. I'll use fear as the primary emotion, but as always, focus on the emotion that is most true to your experience.

Karate Chop *(Repeat 3 times)*: Even though it scares me so much that he has allergies/asthma, I deeply and completely love and accept myself.

Eyebrow: All this fear

Side of Eye: So much anxiety

Under Eye: These allergies/asthma attacks

Under Nose: So stressful

Under Mouth: I feel so helpless

Collarbone: All this fear that I can't make them stop

Under Arm: So much anxiety

Top of Head: All this fear

Eyebrow: I can't relax

Side of Eye: Always trying to prevent symptoms

Under Eye: It's so scary

Under Nose: And so stressful

Under Mouth: I feel exhausted by it

Collarbone: But I need this stress to stay alert

Under Arm: It wears me out, though

Top of Head: Maybe I can let it go

Eyebrow: Letting myself feel the stress now

Side of Eye: And releasing it

Under Eye: Letting it go from every cell in my body now

Under Nose: I don't need this stress to be alert

Under Mouth: I can relax now

Collarbone: Allowing myself to feel safe

Under Arm: Letting go of this stress now

Top of Head: Feeling safe and relaxed in my body now

Take a deep breath, and rate the intensity of your emotion now. Continue Tapping until you get the desired relief.

Next let's look at how to use Tapping with your child on their allergies and asthma.

Note: As always, when Tapping with your child, tailor your words to your child's age and experience.

Overcoming Allergies and Asthma

At 14 years old, Angie was sad, angry and frustrated about her ongoing struggle with food allergies and asthma. More often than not, the food her friends ate near her would cause her to wake up with her face swollen and eyes puffy.

Her allergic reactions were also often accompanied by asthma attacks, as well as persistent coughing. Typically, these symptoms would last for several days before finally tapering off. The experience was miserable and stressful.

Like most kids, Angie just wanted to be like everyone else.

After years of stress and suffering, Angie began Tapping with the help and guidance of her mother. They tapped through her allergy and asthma symptoms, her emotions around being different, as well as her fear of becoming "ugly" when her symptoms flared up.

Within a couple of months, Angie's entire life began to change. She quickly began to feel better. Within six months of Tapping, all of Angie's food allergies and asthma disappeared completely. She can now eat all different kinds of foods without experiencing any symptoms.

This story is a great reminder of how closely connected our emotional, physical and mental health all are. Using Tapping, Angie was able to address all of these components of wellness at the same time, which paved the way for her to heal fully in a fairly short period of time.

The even better news is that Angie's progress didn't stop there. Since resolving her allergies and asthma, she has continued to use Tapping on other challenges, including anxiety around math, resistance to homework and difficult teachers. As a result, she's overcome obstacles with relative ease, and feels more confident and fearless than ever before.

In the next section, we'll look at Tapping on asthma. For now, let's look at how you can use Tapping with your child when allergies flare up. If, like Angie, your child experiences both simultaneously, feel free to incorporate asthma into this Tapping script.

Child Tapping: Overcoming Allergies

In this Tapping script we'll focus on food allergies. If your child's allergies are triggered by pollen or some other irritant, make sure to change the words to reflect his/her experience.

First have your child share how they feel about their allergies. Are they angry, frustrated, sad or anxious? If you can, focus on their primary emotion. Then ask them to measure the intensity of that emotion on a scale of 0 to 10 or using the "this much" method of measurement.

Take a deep breath and begin by Tapping 3 times on the Karate Chop point.

Karate Chop *(Repeat 3 times)*: Even though I'm so frustrated, angry and sad about my allergies, I'm a great kid and I'm okay.

Eyebrow: These allergies

Side of Eye: They make me so mad!

Under Eye: So frustrated that they won't go away

Under Nose: So sad that I have to be so careful about what I eat

Under Mouth: Why can't I eat what my friends are eating?

Collarbone: It's not fair!

Under Arm: So mad about these allergies

Top of Head: So sick of not being able to eat like my friends

Eyebrow: Really mad about these allergies

Side of Eye: I want them to go away

Under Eye: Hate how they make me feel and how they make me look

Under Nose: But I'm still a great kid

Under Mouth: It's okay for me to feel mad, sad and frustrated about my allergies

Collarbone: It's safe to feel all of this

Under Arm: And it's safe to let these feelings go

Top of Head: I can relax now

Eyebrow: And feel safe in my body

Side of Eye: I'm a great kid!

Under Eye: I can relax now

Under Nose: I can feel safe in my body

Under Mouth: I can feel safe around food

Collarbone: Letting myself feel safe and quiet now

Under Arm: I'm a great kid!

Top of Head: And I'm okay

Take a deep breath and check in again on the intensity of your child's primary emotion. Keep Tapping until they get the desired relief.

Quieting an Asthma Attack

For the previous ten years, Kris had lived in fear of her son's asthma attacks. She'd tried multiple inhalers over several years, but none had worked. Each time an attack began, her son's body would go limp in her arms as he gasped for air and his face turned blue. While the ambulance had always arrived in time, each experience was traumatic.

One day, just as an asthma attack was beginning, Kris began Tapping on him. Almost immediately, his attack halted, and very quickly he was able to breathe normally again. From that point forward, Kris began using it with both of her children.

Child Tapping: Quieting an Asthma Attack

If you haven't yet tapped with your child, don't wait until their next asthma attack to try it. Instead, try leading them through some rounds of Tapping when they're nervous or anxious about something, including having an asthma attack.

For instance, if you're undertaking an activity, like taking a family hike, that has caused them to have an asthma attack in the past, you could do some rounds of Tapping to relieve their anxiety about having an asthma attack on this hike, too.

To do that, first have them rate their nervousness or anxiety on a scale of 0 to 10 or by extending their arms and using the "this much" method of measurement.

Then begin by Tapping 3 times on the Karate Chop point:

Karate Chop *(Repeat 3 times)*: Even though I'm so nervous about having another asthma attack, I'm a great kid and I'm okay!

Eyebrow: So scared

Side of Eye: I don't want to have another asthma attack

Under Eye: It's so scary when it happens

Under Nose: I can't breathe

Under Mouth: I'm scared it will happen again

Collarbone: That's okay

Under Arm: Everything's okay

Top of Head: And I'll be okay

Eyebrow: I'm a great kid!

Side of Eye: I can stop worrying now

Under Eye: I'm an awesome kid

Under Nose: And I can breathe great!

Under Mouth: I'm a great kid!

Collarbone: And everything's okay

Under Arm: I can feel good now

Top of Head: I can breathe great

Eyebrow: I'm an awesome kid

Side of Eye: And I can stop worrying now

Under Eye: I can breathe great!

Under Nose: I can trust my body to breathe

Under Mouth: I can let the air flow easily now

Collarbone: Letting air flow easily through my lungs

Under Arm: I can breathe easily and naturally

Top of Head: I can feel safe and trust that I'm okay

Have your child rate their nervousness or anxiety now. Keep Tapping until they get the desired relief.

If you're using Tapping at the start of an asthma attack, keep it simple:

- Skip the rating step, and begin Tapping on the points on their body for them.

- Beginning on the Eyebrow point, tap through the points on your child. If you're only able to get to one or two points on their body, that's fine, just keep Tapping on as many points as you can.

- If it helps them, you can use soothing statements as you tap on the points, such as:

  - "Releasing this stress now"
  - "Clearing the airways"
  - "I can relax and breathe freely now"
  - "Letting air pass through my airways easily"
  - "I can relax and breathe easily now"

Quieting Anxiety Caused by Asthma

Julie didn't seem to be herself. A 1st grader, she'd suddenly begun having extreme tantrums every morning about not wanting to go to school. Julie's resistance had gotten so extreme, in fact, that she was fighting the school principal every morning. She hadn't done this in kindergarten, and her parents were worried, and also unsure about how to help their daughter.

Overcome with worry, Julie's mother called the school counselor in tears one day. "I really need your help," she said. "I don't know what else to do." The counselor, who uses Tapping with children often, set up a meeting with both of Julie's parents and explained Tapping.

During the meeting, her parents explained that Julie suffers from severe asthma. They'd been to the emergency room several times as a result. During the most recent visit, the ER doctor had told them that that particular attack had likely been a panic attack, rather than asthma.

With Julie's parents' permission, the counselor called Julie into their meeting. They spent some time talking about what was happening, and asked if Julie would be willing to try Tapping. Once Julie felt comfortable, her parents left the room.

Once Julie had learned the Tapping points, Julie shared that her anxiety about being at school was a 10 out of 10. She explained, "I don't know why, but I don't want to leave my mom." While Tapping, she then shared the story of her last asthma attack, and how scary it was not being able to breathe. Her anxiety went down to an 8 out of 10.

The counselor then asked her how she felt when she had to separate from her mom every morning at school. Julie shared that she was terrified that she wouldn't be able to breathe at school, and that caused her to panic. Continuing to tap through the points, Julie focused on several aspects of her anxiety about leaving her mom:

- What if something happens to me?
- I can't breathe.
- What will happen at school if I can't breathe?
- I have my inhaler at school.
- I would want my mom.

Julie's anxiety then went down to a 5 out of 10. They then continued to tap, using the setup statement:

"Even though I have this fear of not being able to breathe, I know I'm safe and I'm a good kid." They followed that with reminder phrases, such as:

- I'm safe.
- I can breathe.
- I'm okay.
- I have my inhaler.
- I'm safe at school.

Julie's anxiety then dropped to a 3 out of 10. The counselor tasked her with homework—to teach her parents how to tap, and to tap for a few minutes each night before bed. During the next couple of weeks, Julie met once a week with the school counselor to discuss and monitor her progress. She then formed a small Tapping group with two girls in the 2nd grade. Julie assumed a leadership role in that group and taught the other girls how to tap. Since then, she continues to meet with her group once a month to check in and maintain their progress, and her own as well.

As a result of her Tapping, Julie's anxiety around going to school has almost completely dissipated to somewhere between 0 and 2 out of 10. She's had no asthma or panic attacks since.

This story is a great demonstration of how interwoven our emotions are with our physical health. Although Julie's anxiety may have begun after her asthma, it became such a part of her condition that Tapping on her anxiety led to profound physical as well as emotional healing.

Child Tapping: Calming Anxiety after an Asthma Attack

Once the attack has passed, you may want to lead them through some Tapping on releasing the trauma they experienced.

When they're ready, have them rate the primary emotion they feel about the attack using either the 0 to 10 scale or the "this much" method.

Next, begin by Tapping 3 times on the Karate Chop point:

Karate Chop *(Repeat 3 times)*: Even though it was so scary not being able to breathe, I'm a great kid and I'm okay.

Eyebrow: So scary

Side of Eye: I couldn't breathe

Under Eye: I want it to stop

Under Nose: Just too scary

Under Mouth: But I'm okay

Collarbone: I'm a great kid!

Under Arm: I don't have to be scared now

Top of Head: I'm okay

Eyebrow: I'm an awesome kid!

Side of Eye: And I'm okay now

Under Eye: I can stop feeling scared

Under Nose: I'm okay now!

Under Mouth: I can feel safe in my body now

Collarbone: I can trust that I'm okay

Under Arm: I'm safe

Top of Head: I can breathe easily

Eyebrow: I'm a great kid!

Side of Eye: And I'm okay

Under Eye: I can breathe easily

Under Nose: I can feel the air going in and out

Under Mouth: I'm breathing easily

Collarbone: I'm safe in my body

Under Arm: It's easy to breathe now

Top of Head: And I'm a great kid!

Have your child rate the emotional intensity of the memory of his or her last asthma attack now. Keep Tapping until s/he gets the desired relief.

TAPPING WITH YOUR CHILD: INJURY HEALING

While Tapping can't fuse broken bones, it does initiate the relaxation response in the body, which is when the body's healing abilities are most powerful.

When using Tapping on injuries, the best way to get immediate results is to tap on the symptoms related to the injury, whether it's physical discomfort, frustration, limited mobility, aching, pain, heat, cold and so on.

If your goal is to promote healing in the body, it's also a good idea to do general Tapping on letting your body relax and heal.

We'll begin by doing that general Tapping on you, and then look at how to tap with your child on his/her injury.

Adult Tapping: Promoting Healing in the Body

Let's first take a look at your beliefs around your body's ability to heal itself. For instance, when you have an injury or wound, do you tell yourself that healing is a slow and painful process, or something your body can do quickly and with minimal discomfort? Similarly, do you believe that your body has an easy or hard time healing itself?

Select one limiting belief you have around your body's ability to heal itself and rate how true it feels on a scale of 0 to 10.

Take a deep breath, then tap on the Karate Chop point:

Karate Chop (*Repeat 3 times*): Even though I don't trust in my body's ability to heal itself, I deeply and completely love and accept myself

Eyebrow: I don't always trust my body

Side of Eye: I'm not always sure it can heal

Under Eye: It's frustrating

Under Nose: I want to feel good and be healthy

Under Mouth: But I'm not always sure my body can heal itself

Collarbone: I know it's supposed to heal itself

Under Arm: But it doesn't always seem to do that

Top of Head: It's stressful to think about

Eyebrow: I want to feel good and be healthy

Side of Eye: I want my body to be able to heal itself

Under Eye: Maybe my stress is getting in the way

Under Nose: I can let that stress go

Under Mouth: I can let my body relax now

Collarbone: And relax my mind

Under Arm: Letting my body and mind relax now

Top of Head: I can relax and let my body heal itself

Eyebrow: I can trust my body to do the healing work

Side of Eye: Letting my body and mind relax completely now

Under Eye: My body can heal itself

Under Nose: I trust in my body to heal itself

Under Mouth: I can relax when I think about that

Collarbone: Feeling peaceful and calm in my body and mind now

Under Arm: Allowing myself to feel total relaxation now

Top of Head: Feeling completely peaceful now

Take a deep breath and rate how true your limiting belief feels now. Keep Tapping until you get the desired relief.

Now let's look at how to tap with your child on allowing his/her body to heal itself.

Note: As always, when Tapping with your child, tailor your words to your child's age and experience.

Regaining Mobility

After spending weeks in a cast to heal her broken arm, Reagan, 10 years old, was relieved and excited to begin regaining movement again. Her doctor had told her it would take two weeks before she'd be able to straighten it fully, but she was anxious to make it happen sooner. Wanting to support her, Reagan's mom offered to do some Tapping with her, provided she didn't force her arm to move if it didn't feel right. Reagan agreed.

They then began Tapping on straightening her arm. By the end of their second round of Tapping, Reagan had fully straightened her arm without having to stress or strain.

Although stories like this can seem like a fluke, there's very real science behind them. As we saw in Chapter 2, stress, along with challenging emotions like anxiety, fear and more, create a very real physiological process in the body known as the stress response. One thing that happens when the body is in this stress response is that excessive amounts of hormones get released into the body, causing muscles to restrict. Over time this tightening can lead to chronic pain, as well as limited mobility.

By Tapping on releasing resistance to moving her arm, Reagan was lowering the amount of stress in her body, and also telling her brain, which initiates the stress response, that it's safe to relax and move her arm.

I've seen results like Reagan's several hundred times during my years of Tapping with people. To this day it's incredible watching people's amazement as their pain or mobility issues vanish before their very eyes.

Child Tapping: Overcoming Injury-Related Physical Symptoms

Since the best way to use Tapping for injury healing is by focusing on a symptom of your child's injury, you first need to find out which physical symptom is bothering him/her. Is a cast causing the injured area to itch? Do they have other injury-related sensations, like heat or cold, throbbing, burning, numbness, sharp pain, or discomfort when they're trying to fall asleep?

Have your child focus on the one injury-related physical symptom that is most bothersome right now. Then ask him/her to rate the intensity of that symptom on a scale of 0 to 10, or using the "this much" method of measurement.

If, due to the injury, your child is unable to access all of the Tapping points, don't be concerned. Get to as many as you can, and feel free to tap on your child for him/her.

I'll use itching as the physical symptom, but of course, substitute your child's symptom and words as you tap. While Tapping, be as specific as you can be about where on his/her body your child is feeling the symptom, and if possible, have him/her describe the sensation.

Karate Chop *(Repeat 3 times)*: Even though I feel this itching, I'm a great kid and I'm okay.

Eyebrow: So Itchy

Side of Eye: It won't stop

Under Eye: All this itching

Under Nose: This itching is bothering me

Under Mouth: It won't stop

Collarbone: All this itching

Under Arm: I want it to stop

Top of Head: That's okay, I can relax anyway

Eyebrow: I can let this itching stop

Side of Eye: I can feel calm in my body now

Under Eye: I can feel quiet in my mind now

Under Nose: Letting this itching go

Under Mouth: Letting myself feel calm now

Collarbone: Letting my body relax

Under Arm: And letting this itching go now

Top of Head: I can feel peaceful now

Eyebrow: I feel quiet and calm in my body now

Side of Eye: Letting any remaining itching feeling go now

Under Eye: I can feel peaceful and quiet in my body and mind now

Under Nose: I can relax and feel calm now

Under Mouth: Comfortable in my own skin

Collarbone: At peace with my body

Under Arm: Feeling peaceful and calm now

Top of Head: Feeling comfortable and calm in my body now

When s/he is ready, have your child rate the intensity of his/her physical sensation now. Keep Tapping until s/he gets the desired relief.

Child Tapping: **Releasing Injury-Related Stress**

In addition to physical symptoms, injury can also cause stress, anxiety, frustration and other challenging emotions. All of these contribute to the amount of stress your child's body is under. To make the healing process both more efficient and more pleasant, you can use Tapping with your child to relieve the emotional stress s/he may be feeling as a result of her/his injury.

First ask your child how s/he is feeling about her/his injury. Is s/he frustrated by the length of time it's taking to heal? Anxious about the pain s/he is experiencing, or about re-injuring her/himself?

Once s/he has shared her/his primary emotion, have her/him rate its intensity on a scale of 0 to 10 or using the "this much" method of measurement. As always, be as specific as possible as you're Tapping.

Let's begin by Tapping on the Karate Chop point:

Karate Chop *(Repeat 3 times)*: Even though I feel all this stress because of this injury, I'm an awesome kid and I'm okay.

Eyebrow: All this stress

Side of Eye: It's because of my injury

Under Eye: So much stress

Under Nose: Because of this injury

Under Mouth: I can let go of this stress

Collarbone: And let my body relax now

Under Arm: Even though I still have this injury

Top of Head: I can feel calm and quiet inside now

Eyebrow: Letting go of this icky feeling about my injury

Side of Eye: Even though I still have this injury

Under Eye: It makes me feel icky

Under Nose: I can let that go now

Under Mouth: I can feel peaceful inside

Collarbone: Even though I still have this boo-boo

Under Arm: I can feel quiet and calm inside

Top of Head: I can stop feeling icky now

Eyebrow: My body has magic powers!

Side of Eye: My body can heal itself!

Under Eye: I can feel quiet and calm inside

Under Nose: And let my body use its magic powers

Under Mouth: I can feel good now

Collarbone: I can feel peaceful now

Under Arm: And let my body use its magic powers

Top of Head: Feeling calm and quiet inside now

Have your child rate his/her stress (or "icky feeling," etc.) on a scale of 0 to 10 or using the "this much" method of measurement. Keep Tapping until s/he gets the desired relief.

TAPPING WITH YOUR CHILD: PAIN RELIEF

My first experience with Tapping was about fifteen years ago when, out of the blue, I began suffering from a stiff neck that remained immobilized for several days. I'd read about "this weird Tapping thing" online, and finally broke down one day and tried it, desperate for relief.

I was thrilled and amazed to discover that after just a few minutes of Tapping I had a working neck again. Since that day, I've worked with thousands of people, using Tapping to relieve temporary as well as long-term chronic pain.

While many of us have been taught that pain is purely physical, there's an extensive body of research connecting our beliefs and emotions with physical sensations, especially pain. While temporary pain—the kind of pain we feel immediately after an injury or cut, for example—is a natural part of the body's healing process, studies have shown that ongoing chronic pain is often tied to repressed emotions like anger, sadness and others.[3]

Whatever the root cause of physical pain at any given instance, the key to alleviating it is quieting the body's stress response. When we let go of that stress, the body defaults to its opposite state, the relaxation response. That's when the body is best able to support pain relief, as well as healing and wellness.

As we've seen, because it sends calming signals directly to the amygdala in the brain, Tapping is a powerful way of putting your body into the relaxation response, and in doing so, relieving pain.

We'll look at some of the ways you can use Tapping with your child on pain s/he is experiencing, but first, let's do some Tapping on the stress and anxiety that your child's pain may create in you.

Adult Tapping: Releasing the Stress of Your Child's Pain

To begin, focus on how your child's pain makes you feel—frustrated, anxious, angry, helpless...? Notice which emotion is most intense for you and rate it on a scale of 0 to 10.

Take a deep breath and begin by Tapping on the Karate Chop point.

Karate Chop *(Repeat 3 times)*: Even though I feel all this stress and <your emotion here> around my child's pain, I deeply and completely love and accept myself.

Eyebrow: I hate that he/she is in pain

Side of Eye: I need to be able to take it away

Under Eye: So stressful watching him/her in pain

Under Nose: I can't stand to watch him/her in all this pain

Under Mouth: It's not right

Collarbone: It's not fair

Under Arm: He/she is too young

Top of Head: So much stress and worry around his/her pain

Eyebrow: This pain

Side of Eye: I'm so frustrated

Under Eye: So angry and stressed about it

Under Nose: I need to be able to take it away

Under Mouth: He/she shouldn't be in so much pain

Collarbone: Too young

Under Arm: It makes me so mad

Top of Head: And so sad

Eyebrow: This pain

Side of Eye: So much stress around it

Under Eye: I can let myself feel it all now

Under Nose: And I can let it go

Under Mouth: All these emotions

Collarbone: I can feel them

Under Arm: And let them go

Top of Head: Feeling safe and relaxed now

Take a deep breath and check back in on the intensity of your primary emotion now. Give it a number and keep Tapping until you get the desired relief.

Now that you've had an experience, let's look at how to use Tapping with your child on the pain they're feeling.

Note: As always, when Tapping with your child, tailor your words to your child's age and experience.

Relieving Pain in Young Cancer Patients

Since September 2007, Deborah Miller, PhD, an EFT practitioner, has volunteered her time and talents to the children's cancer ward at Hospital General Dr. Aurelio Valdivieso in Oaxaca, Mexico.

Known as the Oaxaca Project, Deborah's work has exposed dozens, if not hundreds, of young cancer patients, their families, and the attending hospital staff to the tremendous emotional, mental, physical and clinical benefits of Tapping.

Head oncologist Dr. Armando Quero Hernández has witnessed the powerful impact Tapping has had on his cancer ward, and most especially, on his patients. "As a result of EFT, I started to see changes: the families less tense, kids more dynamic, more comfortable," he explains.

By improving patients' emotional states, Tapping also appears to facilitate immune function, including relieving pain. As a result of those improvements, even terminal cancer patients often require less pain medication. When Tapping is used on an ongoing basis, Dr. Hernández has also seen decreased infections and reduced complications, as well.

The incredible, heartwarming transformations that Tapping produces in kids like these who are facing intense physical, mental and emotional challenges at such young and tender ages is one of the true highlights of the EFT community. By giving kids relief from physical pain, as well as a sense of inner peace, EFT is truly changing the future of our world.

If your child suffers from chronic pain, whether due to disease, illness, an injury, or even unknown causes, know that there are several ways to use Tapping to find relief. In this section, we'll look at a few of the main techniques.

Child Tapping: Relieving Physical Pain

This Tapping exercise can be used for short-term pain from a simple fall or scrape, as well as chronic pain.

First have your child describe the location and nature of his/her pain:

- Where in your body do you feel pain most intensely? (If there are several spots, start by focusing only on the most intense one.)
- Is it a throbbing, stabbing, burning or tingling pain? Describe the pain.
- Does your pain feel hot, cold or neither?
- What color is your pain?
- Does your pain have a shape or texture? If so, describe it.

"Seeing" the pain can help your child to focus on his/her pain, and also brings in more of their senses, which is helpful with Tapping.

Ask your child to rate the intensity of his/her pain on a scale of 0 to 10 or using the "this much" method of measurement.

Take a deep breath and then start by Tapping on the Karate Chop point.

Karate Chop (*Repeat 3 times*): Even though I have this <describe the nature their pain here> in my <location of pain here>, I'm a great kid and I'm okay.

Eyebrow: This <describe pain>

Side of Eye: I can feel it in my <pain location>

Under Eye: It hurts

Under Nose: This <describe pain>

Under Mouth: I can feel it in my <pain location>

Collarbone: It feels so yucky

Under Arm: This <describe pain> in my <pain location>

Top of Head: I want it to go away

Eyebrow: I don't like this pain

Side of Eye: I can put my pain in a bubble

Under Eye: I can let go of my pain bubble

Under Nose: And let it float away

Under Mouth: Bye-bye pain

Collarbone: You can float away now

Under Arm: I can feel calm in my body now

Top of Head: My pain bubble is floating away

Eyebrow: Bye-bye, pain

Side of Eye: You can go away now

Under Eye: I can feel quiet and calm in my body

Under Nose: Bye-bye, pain

Under Mouth: I can feel comfortable in my body now

Collarbone: I can feel calm now

Under Arm: I can feel quiet inside now

Top of Head: Feeling calm and happy in my body now

Take a deep breath, and have your child rate his/her pain again. Keep Tapping until s/he gets the desired relief.

CHASING THE PAIN

While Tapping on physical pain, people sometimes experience a shift. The pain may move to a new location or change in some way. For example, after Tapping on a stabbing pain in your lower back, you may feel a new pain radiating up and down your spine. Tapping through these shifts is a process that's referred to as "chasing the pain." If this happens, keep Tapping until your pain is gone or you get the desired relief. These shifts are a positive sign that your body is responding to Tapping.

If Tapping on the pain sensation(s) doesn't provide sufficient relief, you can look at other related aspects, including events. Let's look at how to do that next.

Child Tapping: Releasing a Pain-Related Event

There are times when pain can be related to an emotionally charged event. If, for instance, your child has pain from a traumatic injury (from a car accident, for example), pain after surgery, or other, you may want to tap with him/her on that event using the "Tell the Story" technique.

A great place to start is with when/where the pain started. If, for instance, your child has been in pain since that car accident, and s/he is willing to tap on those memories, begin by Tapping through what s/he remembers.

Whether the event happened 10 minutes or two years ago, have your child recall it and rate the intensity of the memory, either on a scale of 0 to 10 or using the "this much" method of measurement.

Then begin Tapping on the Karate Chop point and continue Tapping through the points as your child tells the story. Gently encourage her or him to recall as many details of the event as possible.

At each point of emotional intensity in the story, have your child pause the story, and rate the intensity of just that moment in the memory. Then tap through just that moment until it's been neutralized.

Progress through the story, pausing to tap through and neutralize each moment of emotional intensity.

Once you've gotten to the end of the story, neutralizing each peak point in the story through Tapping, have your child begin telling the story again. If s/he still experiences an emotional charge at any peak points in the story, pause and tap to neutralize those moments.

Once your child can tell the entire story from beginning to end without experiencing an emotional charge, you've successfully neutralized the entire event.

To complete your Tapping, you can then lead your child through some positive rounds of Tapping on releasing the pain:

Karate Chop: I can feel relaxed in my body
Karate Chop: I can feel safe with this memory now
Karate Chop: This pain was keeping me safe

Eyebrow: But I'm safe now

Side of Eye: I can let go of this pain for good

Under Eye: I can feel safe in my body now

Under Nose: I can let this pain go

Under Mouth: My body can relax now

Collarbone: I'm safe in my body

Under Arm: I'm a great kid

Top of Head: And I'm okay!

Eyebrow: I can feel comfortable in my body now

Side of Eye: My body can feel good now!

Under Eye: I'm safe in my body

Under Nose: I can feel good now

Under Mouth: I'm a great kid!

Collarbone: And I'm okay

Under Arm: I can let my body feel quiet inside

Top of Head: And I can feel quiet inside

Eyebrow: I'm a great kid!

Side of Eye: And I'm okay

Under Eye: I can let my body heal

Under Nose: I can let my body feel good now

Under Mouth: I'm a great kid!

Collarbone: I'm safe

Under Arm: And I can feel good!

Top of Head: I'm a great kid and I'm okay!

Take a deep breath together and have your child rate his/her pain again. Keep Tapping until s/he gets the desired relief.

RELIEVING CHRONIC PAIN WITH TAPPING

Some of the first documented research findings around the science of physical pain and our emotions came out of the National Institute of Health (NIH) in the 1980s. That field of study has since continued, advanced by the pioneering work done at Stanford University and beyond. It's such an important topic, in fact, that I wrote an entire book on it! Check out *The Tapping Solution for Pain Relief* for complete details, as well as a full-length program on how to use Tapping to relieve chronic pain.

Child Tapping: Releasing the Emotions behind the Pain

Since research has shown that physical pain, especially when it's chronic, can be linked to repressed emotion, many people also experience relief by Tapping on the emotion(s) behind the pain.

Begin by asking your child questions like:

- When you think about your pain, how do you feel? Sad? Frustrated? Mad?

- If your pain were an emotion, what emotion would it be?

If it helps, you can also have your child draw a picture of his or her pain and then tell you about the picture. You can then ask your child how that pain feels:

- Is that pain mad?

- Is it sad or frustrated?

- What does your pain want to say?

As always, use your child's answers as you tap. For instance, if your child's pain is mad because it hurts too much to go play outside, your Tapping might look something like this:

Karate Chop *(Repeat 3 times)*: Even though I have this pain and I'm mad about not being able to go outside and play, I'm a great kid and I'm okay.

Eyebrow: This pain

Side of Eye: This pain is mad

Under Eye: This pain means I can't play outside

Under Nose: This pain is so mad

Under Mouth: I want to play outside

Collarbone: And this pain is so mad that I can't

Under Arm: It hurts too much

Top of Head: This mad pain

Eyebrow: This icky, yucky pain

Side of Eye: It's mad

Under Eye: It wants to play outside

Under Nose: This mad pain

Under Mouth: It's so mad!

Collarbone: And it hurts so much!

Under Arm: I can let it be mad

Top of Head: I can let it be *really* mad

Eyebrow: It's okay if this pain is mad

Side of Eye: I can let it be mad

Under Eye: And now I can let it be happy!

Under Nose: I can let it feel better

Under Mouth: I can let it feel safe and quiet

Collarbone: Letting go of this mad pain

Under Arm: Turning into it a happy feeling

Top of Head: Letting my body feel happy and free now!

Take a deep breath together and have your child rate his or her pain again, as well as the emotion that's linked to the pain. If the pain or the emotion behind the pain has shifted, tap on that new experience. Keep Tapping until your child gets the desired relief.

ADDENDUM

Tapping in Schools

Bringing children of different ages, backgrounds and skill levels into a single environment where they need to learn and develop social/emotional skills while also meeting pre-set academic standards is a daunting challenge, at best. It's no surprise, then, that the need for Tapping is often most evident within the school environment.

Through The Tapping Solution Foundation, we've had the incredible honor and privilege of introducing Tapping to schools around the country. Each and every time, it's deeply inspiring to watch students and faculty alike benefit from the quick stress relief and relaxing effects they experience. We've noticed that teachers often find that the few minutes of Tapping they do in the classroom saves them time throughout the remainder of the day, since students are often calmer and more attentive once they've tapped.

Whether you're a parent hoping to introduce Tapping to your child's school, or a teacher or faculty member wanting to use Tapping in school, I'm thrilled to share our online resources on how to bring Tapping into your own or your child's school.

First, though, let me share a few of the many success stories around Tapping in schools.

Tapping in Elementary School

A mother of two, Kelly was excited about introducing mindfulness to her son's 2nd grade class. Over a six-month period, she came in periodically and taught the kids how to tap, as well as different ways to use grounding meditation. The kids quickly got excited about Tapping and began requesting to do more Tapping every time she came to their classroom.

Noticing how much the class was enjoying Tapping, Kelly asked her son to help her rewrite an adult Tapping meditation specifically for him and his classmates. During that meditation, while the kids tapped through the points, they were asked to visualize a time when they'd had a painful or hurtful experience. They then mentally placed the memory inside a bubble. As they tapped, they were asked to release that bubble. A few of the children told Kelly afterward that during that exercise they'd released hurt feelings that they'd felt since preschool.

Each time they tapped together as a group, Kelly made sure to end their Tapping with a few rounds about what they liked and appreciated about themselves and each other.

Seeing how much Tapping was helping her class to focus, the teacher applied for permission to lead the mindfulness and Tapping class herself when Kelly's volunteer months were over!

I've been told by numerous teachers and school administrators that elementary school is an especially good time to introduce children to Tapping. At these ages, children are generally open to trying new things and less likely to feel scrutinized socially. As a result, they're often more open to trying this "weird Tapping thing." Keeping the practice fun and game-like is, of course, especially important during these early years.

Tapping in Middle & High School

Older children, both middle- and high-school-aged, also benefit enormously from Tapping. Since by this age social pressures and the urge to rebel are more prominent, the key here is to introduce Tapping in a way that's tailored to their age and current challenges. For Beverly, a teacher and Tapping specialist, that meant solving an immediate and urgent issue in a classroom she was visiting one day.

During a typical week, Beverly travels to as many as six different schools in her district, sometimes working with groups of students in classrooms, and at other times with individual students on specific issues. On this particular day, she arrived at one of the classrooms that had students suffering from emotional disturbances and found that a student was in the midst of a rage-fueled meltdown. He'd begun throwing chairs, pushing tables and screaming at his classmates and teachers. Since all of the children in that class suffer from emotional disturbances already, it was imperative that he be removed from the classroom quickly.

Once Beverly had gotten him out into the hall, he continued to rant, but also mentioned that he hadn't slept well the night before. There had been a major disturbance at home. Something had happened with his mom and the neighborhood where they live.

Beverly immediately asked him if he'd be willing to do some Tapping. He said yes, and began Tapping along, repeating her setup statement about the difficult night he'd had. Within a few minutes of Tapping, he was completely calm. He asked Beverly if he could go back into the classroom to apologize to his teacher.

When they re-entered the room, his teacher was working at a table with several other students. He silently walked over to her, gently took her hand, and bent forward to ask her if she'd accept his apology. He explained that he'd had a terrible night, but was really sorry for how he'd behaved. His teacher gratefully accepted the apology, and expressed her sorrow about his night. She then offered to tap with him if he ever felt like that again.

Before I share our online resources on how to bring Tapping into schools, let's look at one more story.

Giving High School Students the Gift of Self-Mastery

Ellen, a school counselor and life coach, was walking down the aisle at the grocery store when a former student suddenly approached and gave her a huge bear hug. Startled by the student's sudden presence, she hesitated, trying to place him. He quickly reminded her that he'd been in the summer class she'd taught at Upward Bound at Sacred Heart University in Fairfield, CT. The class was titled *Brain Hacking*. "It was the best thing I did all summer! One of the best classes I've ever taken!" the student exclaimed.

Brain Hacking had been a new experience for her and her students. It was also the first time she'd added Tapping to the curriculum. The class had begun with research about the brain, focusing on discoveries about neuroplasticity. Realizing that they could change their brains excited and intrigued the students.

As the class progressed, they got even more excited about the difference between the brain and the mind. They also learned about the brain's alarm system, how we respond to stress, recover from shame or a poor decision, and stay healthy during emergencies and other challenging times.

Once they'd gained a better understanding about how the brain is affected by emotions and behavior, Ellen taught them how to use Tapping. It's often a tough sell to high school students, who are typically focused on being "cool" and fitting in. In spite of Tapping's "weird" factor, however, the students were so excited about the possibility of transforming their brains that they were eager to try it. Before long, Tapping became one of their favorite parts of the class.

For the final class project, several students made Tapping a central focus of their final projects. One girl even wrote and performed spoken word poetry that emphasized how much Tapping had helped her.

When I asked Ellen why she felt she'd had success with this notoriously challenging age group, she shared that she'd challenged the students to be curious about their brains. In doing so, she'd appealed to their individuality in a uniquely powerful and age-appropriate way.

How to Get Tapping into Your School

For a practice that's so tied to self-acceptance, Tapping has had to face some fairly significant hurdles in being accepted into education's mainstream curriculum. Fortunately, that is changing, often thanks to state and/or district-level Health & Wellness requirements for students.

Given the magnitude and ever-changing nature of school regulations and requirements, The Tapping Solution Foundation is offering multiple free online resources to support parents, teachers and school staff who want to bring Tapping into their schools.

For complete information, including summary sheets about the science behind Tapping, as well as sample letters that you're welcome to use and edit to meet your needs, please visit The Tapping Solution Foundation at http://www.tappingsolutionfoundation.org/tapping-teachers-students/.

Endnotes

Chapter 1

1. R.A. Clay, "Stressed in America," American Psychological Association, January 2011, Vol. 42, No. 1, http://www.apa.org/monitor/2011/01/stressed-america.aspx

2. Marian Wilde, "Are we stressing out our kids?," December 16, 2016, http://www.greatschools.org/gk/articles/stressed-out-kids/

3. Stephanie Liou, "Neuroplasticity," Huntington's Outreach Project for Education, at Stanford, June 26, 2010, http://web.stanford.edu/group/hopes/cgi-bin/hopes_test/neuroplasticity/

4. Rick Hanson, PhD, *Hardwiring Happiness*, Harmony/Random House, October 8, 2013

5. Ibid.

6. Dawson Church, PhD, "EFT Lowers Stress Hormones," Foundation for Epigenetic Medicine, Santa Rosa, CA, January 2011, http://www.eftuniverse.com/eft-related-press-releases/study-finds-eft-tapping-lowers-cortisol-significantly

7. David Milbradt, LAc, "Bonghan Channels in Acupuncture," Acupuncture Today, April, 2009, Vol. 10, Issue 04, http://acupuncturetoday.com/mpacms/at/article.php?id=31918

Chapter 3

1. "Stress in America findings," American Psychological Association, November 9, 2010, https://www.apa.org/news/press/releases/stress/2010/national-report.pdf

2. James Clear, "The Theory of Cumulative Stress: How to Recover When Stress Builds Up," https://jamesclear.com/cumulative-stress

3. "Stress in America findings," American Psychological Association, November 9, 2010, https://www.apa.org/news/press/releases/stress/2010/national-report.pdf

4. Christiane Northrup, MD, *Goddesses Never Age: The Secret Prescription for Radiance, Vitality, and Well-Being*, Hay House, February 24, 2015

5. Katy Steinmetz, "Help! My Parents Are Millennials," *Time*, October 26, 2015, Vol. 186, No. 17, pp 38-43

Chapter 4

1. Brené Brown, "The Fast Track to Genuine Joy," http://www.oprah.com/spirit/Catastrophizing-How-to-Feel-Joy-Without-Fear

Chapter 10

1. John E. Sarno, *The Divided Mind: The Epidemic of Mindbody Disorders*, Harper Perennial, March 27, 2007

2. "Anxiety and Depression in Children," Anxiety and Depression Association of America, http://www.adaa.org/living-with-anxiety/children/anxiety-and-depression

3. Marina Krakovsky, "Why Feelings of Guilt May Signal Leadership Potential," Stanford Graduate School of Business, April 13, 2012 https://www.gsb.stanford.edu/insights/why-feelings-guilt-may-signal-leadership-potential

Chapter 12

1. "What Is Bullying," stopbullying.gov, http://www.stopbullying.gov/what-is-bullying/definition/index.html

Chapter 14

1. Karen Brown, "What Makes a Resilient Mind," PBS.org, January 14, 2015, http://www.pbs.org/wgbh/nova/next/body/mental-resilience/

Chapter 15

1. https://news.google.com/newspapers?id=idMpAAAAIBAJ&sjid=CQAEAAAAIBAJ&pg=5733%2C524477

2. Mark Hyman, *The UltraMind Solution: Fix Your Broken Brain by Healing Your Body First - The Simple Way to Defeat Depression, Overcome Anxiety, and Sharpen Your Mind*, Scribner, December 20, 2008

3. John E. Sarno, *The Divided Mind: The Epidemic of Mindbody Disorders*, Harper Perennial, March 27, 2007

Index

Y

Acknowledgments

First and foremost, Wyndham, your tireless research and writing on this book is what made it all possible. I know it's taken a long time to get out there, but it was worth the wait! Thank you! Thank you!

To all the parents and educators who shared their incredible stories for this book, I am so grateful for your spreading of Tapping into the world.

To my family and dearest friends, Mom, Dad, Alex, Jess, Karen, Lucas, Malakai, Lucas #2, Olivia… thank you for your support in letting me thrive and contribute to the world. You all truly make this work possible.

To all the wonderful people at Hay House, The Tapping Solution and The Tapping Solution Foundation, whose collaborative efforts have brought this book step-by-step into the world, thank you! A special shout-out to Alison Partridge, who combed through it many times to make it the best book possible, and who likes to see her name here. :) Oh, and Allison Price Taylor, might as well get you in here now. Hey! Deb and Scott too, hey! Good enough?

To my wife, Brenna, who makes me a better parent every day and is the best mom in the world; and most of all, because this book is really for the kids, to my little munchkin, June, and any future munchkins to come. You light up my life!

About the Author

Nicolas Ortner is the Founder and CEO of The Tapping Solution, LLC. He has been a leader in the movement to introduce Emotional Freedom Techniques (EFT), an innovative self-care method of healing, into the mainstream.

EFT, also known as Tapping, is a simple, effective, natural healing method that combines ancient Chinese acupressure and modern psychology. Nick has shared this powerful technique with millions of people, helping them to connect with their unique potential, take control of their personal health and healing, and manifest happy, productive, abundant lives.

Nick is also the *New York Times* best-selling author of *The Tapping Solution: A Revolutionary System for Stress-Free Living* and *The Tapping Solution for Pain Relief: A Step-by-Step Guide to Reducing and Eliminating Chronic Pain.*

Nick's newest book, *The Tapping Solution for Manifesting Your Greatest Self: 21 Days to Releasing Self-Doubt, Cultivating Inner Peace, and Creating a Life You Love,* guides readers through a 21-day process of self-discovery and self-development. He has also produced first-of-their-kind online programs that teach easy, effective ways to apply Tapping to anything limiting a person's life or health.

Nick lives in Newtown, Connecticut with his wife, Brenna, and daughter, June. Follow Nick at Facebook.com/Nortner, Twitter@NickOrtner or Instagram @nickortner.

Hay House Titles of Related Interest

YOU CAN HEAL YOUR LIFE, the movie, starring Louise Hay & Friends
(available as a 1-DVD program, an expanded 2-DVD set, and an online streaming video)
Learn more at www.hayhouse.com/louise-movie

THE SHIFT, the movie,
starring Dr. Wayne W. Dyer
(available as a 1-DVD program, an expanded 2-DVD set, and an online streaming video)
Learn more at www.hayhouse.com/the-shift-movie

• • •

Gorilla Thumps and Bear Hugs: A Tapping Solution Children's Story,
by Alex Ortner and Erin Mariano

The Tapping Solution for Teenage Girls: How to Stop Freaking Out and Keep Being Awesome,
by Christine Wheeler

The Tapping Solution for Weight Loss and Body Confidence: A Woman's Guide to Stressing Less, Weighing Less, and Loving More, by Jessica Ortner

All of the above are available at your local bookstore,
or may be ordered by contacting Hay House (see next page).

• • •

We hope you enjoyed this Hay House book. If you'd like to receive
our online catalog featuring additional information on Hay House
books and products, or if you'd like to find out more about the
Hay Foundation, please contact:

Hay House, Inc., P.O. Box 5100, Carlsbad, CA 92018-5100
(760) 431-7695 or (800) 654-5126
(760) 431-6948 (fax) or (800) 650-5115 (fax)
www.hayhouse.com® • www.hayfoundation.org

———

Published and distributed in Australia by:
Hay House Australia Pty. Ltd., 18/36 Ralph St., Alexandria NSW 2015
Phone: 612-9669-4299 • *Fax:* 612-9669-4144 • www.hayhouse.com.au

Published and distributed in the United Kingdom by:
Hay House UK, Ltd., Astley House, 33 Notting Hill Gate, London W11 3JQ
Phone: 44-20-3675-2450 • *Fax:* 44-20-3675-2451 • www.hayhouse.co.uk

Published in India by: Hay House Publishers India,
Muskaan Complex, Plot No. 3, B-2, Vasant Kunj, New Delhi 110 070
Phone: 91-11-4176-1620 • *Fax:* 91-11-4176-1630 • www.hayhouse.co.in

Distributed in Canada by:
Raincoast Books, 2440 Viking Way, Richmond, B.C. V6V 1N2
Phone: 1-800-663-5714 • *Fax:* 1-800-565-3770 • www.raincoast.com

———

Access New Knowledge.
Anytime. Anywhere.

Learn and evolve at your own pace
with the world's leading experts.

www.hayhouseU.com